PRAISE FOR *THE POWER OF*

"Master Stephen Co has helped me
urge you to pay close attention. This bo
—Wayne Dyer, PhD, bestsellin̲g̲ ̲a̲u̲t̲h̲o̲r̲ ̲o̲f̲ *The Power of Intention*

"*The Power of Prana* addresses the very root system of health. When our culture realizes the connection between our emotions and our life energy, then our medical system will change."
—Christiane Northrup, MD, author of the New York Times bestsellers
Women's Bodies, Women's Wisdom and *The Wisdom of Menopause*

"*The Power of Prana* is a compelling bridge between the reader and higher level practices to revitalize your life force!"
—Deepak Chopra, bestselling author of 55 books, including
Peace Is the Way

"Master Stephen Co's *The Power of Prana* makes it easy for people to read and understand esoteric Eastern wisdom on increasing their own energy. The exercises are designed for someone to get the maximum benefit in the least amount of time."
—John Gray, author of *Men Are from Mars, Women Are from Venus*

"This book brilliantly weaves together the practical 'how-to' of doing this very simple pranic breathing routine with a fascinating history of how the inner teachings of the Nine Energizing Breaths became revealed to the world. Master Co is just as good at explaining the teachings in a book as he is at teaching them to his classes. I highly recommend *The Power of Prana*."
—Jack Canfield, coauthor of the *Chicken Soup for the Soul* series

"*The Power of Prana* is elegant, simple, and straightforward in its treatment of the body's energetic anatomy and how we can take steps to increase our personal supply of energy."
—Gay Hendricks, PhD, author of *Conscious Breathing*

"This is a wonderful guide to self healing with energy techniques. Both beginners and advanced students will gain from reading this book and practicing these exercises. As we collectively shift from seeking healing through seeing experts into self healing work—this type of information is becoming more and more important. Whatever your practice and belief system—I recommend you read this book and add some of these practices to your daily energy practice to clear and augment your own body's healing and energy flow."

—Dr. Ann Marie Chiasson, Arizona Center for Integrative Medicine, University of Arizona, Tucson, Arizona.

"Master Co is helping so many people experience deep and lasting happiness. He is one of my 'happiness heroes.' And he has blessed me and the world with his wonderful gifts of healing, love, and light."

—Marci Shimhoff, author of *Happy for No Reason: 7 Steps to Being Happy from the Inside Out* and *Chicken Soup for the Woman's Soul*

"Master Co is a 'teacher who is living his teaching.' He spends his days 24/7 in service to humanity. In this day and age where anything can happen at any moment, knowledge from a great Master on how to enhance and sustain ones energy is a blessing for us all."

—Janet Bray Attwood, author of *The Passion Test*

"*The Power of Prana* shares the age-old wisdom of strengthening the body by properly breathing in and circulating life-force energy. With straightforward illustrations, practicing the powerful breathing techniques is quick, easy, and effective—a perfect start to your day. Prana is all around us and this book teaches you how to harness it in your body. If you follow the simple instructions along with Master Stephen Co's healthy lifestyle suggestions, you will surely create more vitality, happiness, and energy in your daily life."

—Jayme Barrett, author of *Feng Shui Your Life*

"There are many books published today that purport to offer 'secrets.' *The Power of Prana* is different. It delivers true ancient wisdom that can be used simply and easily in the modern world. If you were picking one book to read, this should be it."

—Dr. Joe Vitale, author of *The Attractor Factor*

"An amazing read! Master Co has put together a powerhouse program of exercises that anyone can use to build up their personal energy. And best of all, it really does take only ten minutes a day!"

—Lisa Nichols, author and star of the movie *The Secret*

"Watching Master Stephen Co teach classes all day long, day after day, provided me the best testimonial to the transforming power of the Nine Energizing Breaths as a technique to invigorate the body with stunning amounts of energy and stamina. I was thrilled to learn that the techniques can even work for someone like me, a paraplegic in a wheelchair for many years. Now, I can't imagine living life without them."

—Bobby Muller, former President, Vietnam Veterans of America

"I first learned of the Tibetan breathing exercises two years ago, but it wasn't until this football season (2010) that I started to make them a part of my daily routine. I believe that these exercises were one of the keys to my successful and healthy season. Prior to this season, I was seriously considering retiring from football, mainly because I had doubts about the ability of my body to endure the physical strain of another football season. Those doubts are gone as I feel I have found a way to keep my body feeling young and healthy. Now, instead of reaching for a bottle of pills, I practice the Nine Energizing Breaths. It is mind blowing that these simple exercises could help me feel so much better. "

—Ricky Williams, Heisman Trophy winner and All-Pro NFL running back, Miami Dolphins

"Once again, I am so grateful to be exposed to the teachings of Master Co and his colleagues. The breathing techniques of Master Co revitalize and awaken clarity in the mind and body and give focus to the day."

—Tom Skerritt, actor

"I have always been very aware of energy healing and the power of yogic breath. Recently my ailing mother was given Master Co's work, and it definitely benefited her. Master Co and Dr. Eric Robins have made knowledge of the Nine Energizing Breaths and other powerful practices accessible to the world in a very easy-to-learn manner."

—Sonu Nigam, Indian singing star

"*The Power of Prana* is a simple and interesting way to investigate how you may influence your own health and well-being."

—Susan Smalley, PhD, author of *Fully Present: The Science, Art, and Practice of Mindfulness*

"*The Power of Prana* is a superfascinating look at powerful and down-to-earth principles to understand a simple ancient truth: we are made of energy and we can heal."

—John Paul DeJoria, entrepreneur and philanthropist; cofounder of John Paul Mitchell Systems and The Patrón Spirits Company

"Breathing is the source of all life, energy, and *qi* in humans. To breathe fully and openly brings us back to our infancy where every breath was full and without caution or fear. Learn to breathe and learn to live better with *The Power of Prana.*"

—Frank Shamrock, mixed martial arts legend and former UFC Middleweight Champion

the
power
of prana

the
power
of prana

BREATHE YOUR WAY
TO HEALTH AND VITALITY

MASTER STEPHEN CO
& ERIC B. ROBINS, MD

with **JOHN MERRYMAN**
authors of *Your Hands Can Heal You*

sounds true
BOULDER, COLORADO

Sounds True, Inc.,
Boulder, Colorado 80306

Cover and book design by Rachael Murray
Printed in Canada

NOTE: You should check with your physician before starting this or any new exercise program or breathing routine. This is especially important if you have any preexisting health conditions, such as high blood pressure, migraines, or heart or lung ailments. **Women who are pregnant or think they might be pregnant should not perform the meditations and should check with their physician before performing any of the breathing or physical exercises.**

The authors are grateful to the following for reprint permissions:

Table 2.1, and Exercises 3.1, 3.4, and 3.5 reprinted with the permission of Free Press, a Division of Simon & Schuster, Inc., from *Your Hands Can Heal You: Pranic Healing Energy Remedies to Boost Vitality and Speed Recovery from Common Health Problems* by Master Stephen Co and Eric B. Robins, MD, with John Merryman. Copyright © 2002 by Stephen Co, Eric B. Robins, MD, and John Merryman. All rights reserved.

Exercises 3.2 and 3.3 reprinted with the permission of Gay Hendricks, PhD.

Library of Congress Cataloging-in-Publication Data
    Co, Stephen.
The power of prana : breathe your way to health and vitality / by Stephen Co and Eric B. Robins, MD, with John Merryman.
    p. cm.
Includes bibliographical references.
ISBN 978-1-60407-440-6 (pbk.) — ISBN 978-1-60407-467-3 (e-book)
1. Healing. 2. Vital force. I. Robins, Eric B. II. Merryman, John. III. Title.
RZ401.C596 2011
613.7'046—dc22
                                                                            2011004844

eBook ISBN: 978-1-60407-467-3
10 9 8 7 6 5 4 3 2

Dedication

To our teacher, Grandmaster Choa Kok Sui, for all the priceless wisdom he imparted to us over the years.

While the Nine Energizing Breaths are said to have been brought to the attention of the Western world by Edwin J. Dingle, the founder of the Mentalphysics organization, they are actually a gift from many spiritual teachers, and Grandmaster Choa is part of a long and ancient lineage of such teachers.

The Nine Energizing Breaths and many other techniques in this book have been taken from Grandmaster Choa's two most significant contributions to the world's body of esoteric knowledge: Pranic Healing and Arhatic Yoga. Pranic Healing is a form of "energy medicine" that teaches people to harness universal life force, or *prana*, to heal themselves and others. Grandmaster Choa spent years researching the root teachings of esoteric systems such as yoga, *chi kung*, Kabbalah, and many other traditions in order to create Pranic Healing, a simple, practical, and effective energy healing system that anyone can learn and use. It includes: Basic Pranic Healing, which teaches people to use white prana—pale, bright, elemental healing energy drawn in through one hand and projected out the other—to remedy simple health problems; Advanced Pranic Healing, which enables students to use colored prana—a variety of shades of prana, each with different healing characteristics—to address more complex or serious health problems; and Pranic Psychotherapy, in which people are taught to remove energetic blocks that are at the root of emotional and psychological problems.

Arhatic Yoga is a comprehensive, multileveled energetic and spiritual system of advanced meditations, purification techniques, and prana-generating exercises. It draws heavily on the inner teachings of various conventional and esoteric spiritual traditions, including Christianity, Taoism, Buddhism, Zoroastrianism, and many others. As part of Grandmaster Choa's advanced instruction, Arhatic Yoga students may also take classes in Pranic Feng Shui, Kriyashakti (the science of materialization), Clairvoyance, and Sexual Alchemy (Tantric Yoga), among others.

We were privileged to have been Grandmaster Choa's personal students, and this is our second book based on his work. We are grateful for the opportunity to be able to help present his priceless teachings to you so that you may use his simple program of exercises to give you the energy you need to live the life that you want.

MASTER STEPHEN CO
ERIC B. ROBINS, MD
JOHN MERRYMAN

Contents

Exercises, Figures, and Tables

Tables

Preface

A few years ago, on one of my very first trips to Chicago to teach Basic Pranic Healing, the first class in Grandmaster Choa Kok Sui's energy healing system, I was told by one of our local senior students that a ninety-two-year-old woman had signed up to take the class. When I heard this, I had two thoughts: first, "Good for her! It's good that anyone of that age has an interest in learning something as unique as Pranic Healing," and, second, "I hope she can keep up with the class."

It was her ability to keep up with us that I was most concerned about. We push the class along at a pretty good pace, and the energy that we generate can occasionally make even strong, healthy people feel a little uncomfortable until they get used to it. I wondered if she would be able to tolerate two full days of practice. However, this particular student laughed and told me not to worry about it. "She'll do just fine," she said. The student then proceeded to tell me the woman's remarkable story. Laura Appelgren had been diagnosed with breast cancer some fifty years earlier, and her physician in the Midwest, where she lived, wanted to perform a mastectomy immediately. For whatever reason, Laura refused to go along with it. She went home to consider her next steps, when she happened to see an ad in a magazine that said, "Knowledge is power. Come and learn to breathe in the desert." The ad was for the Institute of Mentalphysics in Southern California. Though her husband urged her to stay and try conventional treatment, she instead took a train west and learned "to breathe in the desert" with the founder of Mentalphysics, Edwin J. Dingle. She practiced the exercises diligently, and after a while, her cancer was completely gone. This experience led her to continue her Mentalphysics breathing practices for the next five decades.

It was clear very quickly in class that I didn't have to worry about Laura's energy or ability to "keep up."

Laura was so full of life that I had her lead the group in many of our stretching and breathing exercises, and she set an amazing pace. She performed her physical movements with precision and briskness, and she breathed with great vigor, inhaling and exhaling audibly.

I found out afterward that when she died a few years later—in her sleep, quietly and serenely—Laura still had all her teeth and did not need glasses. She was an amazing person—physically vigorous, mentally sharp, and full of life until the very end. She attributed it all to her Mentalphysics work and "learning to breathe."

In this book, you are being given the same opportunity to "learn to breathe" that Laura Appelgren was given, the same opportunity she used not only to defeat cancer but also to live robustly into her midnineties. There is one difference, though: the Nine Energizing Breaths you'll learn in this book are the same basic ones practiced by Laura Appelgren, but they've been enhanced to make them even easier to perform, less time-consuming, and even more revitalizing than the original routine she used.

The Nine Energizing Breaths were reportedly introduced to the West by Laura's teacher, Edwin J. Dingle (also known as Ding Le Mei), a British cartographer who learned the exercises in the early part of this century while traveling in Tibet. The exercises are part of a larger body of esoteric knowledge shared by many spiritual teachers, including my teacher, Grandmaster Choa Kok Sui, who developed the systems of Pranic Healing (energy healing) and Arhatic Yoga (a synthesis of yogas). It was Grandmaster Choa who made the simple changes that greatly enhance the intrinsic energy generation and rejuvenation capability of these powerful exercises and make them even easier to perform. The result: the original hour-long exercises have been transformed into a ten-minute routine, even while making them more powerful.

I had the privilege to be a student of Grandmaster Choa for two decades, and to teach his Pranic Healing and Arhatic Yoga courses, as well as the Nine Energizing Breaths. I use the routine myself, and I've taught it to thousands of students. I can personally attest that these exercises will supercharge your energy, your health, and your life. You will be revitalized

IN LIGHT AND LOVE,
MASTER STEPHEN CO

Acknowledgments

My deepest gratitude to: Divine Providence and the Great Ones, whose boundless love and blessings make everything possible. My beloved and respected teacher, Grandmaster Choa Kok Sui, for his love, priceless teachings, blessings, and patience, and especially for giving me the opportunity to serve. Dr. Edwin J. Dingle (Ding Le Mei), for being a powerful instrument in bringing the teachings of Mentalphysics to the West. All my other teachers, for my early years of learning and nurturing. My parents, for bringing me into this world and for the sacrifices they have made to give me a good education and upbringing. My wife, Daphne, and my two lovely daughters, Genevie and Helena, for their continuous support and understanding, and especially for the sacrifices they have made to bring me to the path of service. Dr. Eric Robins and John Merryman, for their expertise, support, and dedication. Karla Alvarez, for enduring the rigorous schedules, deadlines, and countless hours of work as my assistant. Marcos Alvarez, Gabriel Cardiell, and Antoinette Vasquez, for their tireless work and support for the whole United States Pranic Healing mission. Chandan Paramewara, for fantastic work in creating and maintaining our websites and online presence, and also for being a very effective Pranic Healing instructor. All Pranic Healing instructors and supporters, for their untiring assistance in moving the Pranic Healing mission forward. All the students who shared their experiences and helped to validate the powerful teachings in this book. Donald and Barbara Waldrop, and Maria Aquino of the Institute of Mentalphysics, for their years of love and support for sharing the priceless teachings of Dr. Edwin J. Dingle. Jennifer Brown and Haven Iverson of Sounds True, for their guidance and help in getting this book to market. Jerry Miner, for his endless miles on the road and for introducing us to Sounds True. Tom Park of Park Productions, for his nationwide promotion of Pranic Healing. Dave Stroud, for his sage counsel throughout. Wayne Seale, for the fantastic photography that makes anyone look good! The entire Pranic Healing family, for their unending dedication to spreading these priceless teachings to alleviate the suffering of humanity. Countless others not mentioned, for their valuable suggestions and contributions.

MASTER STEPHEN CO

I have many people to thank for helping this book reach fruition. First and foremost is Grandmaster Choa, who had the wonderful ability to find the practical essence of any problem or technique, and who was then able to simplify it into an easy-to-use yet powerful method that could be used to heal the world. What impressed me most about Grandmaster Choa is the degree to which he had refined his character to be a being of unconditional love, patience, and generosity. To Master Stephen Co, my friend and teacher, who is probably one of the most highly developed yogis in the world, and who is living a life of absolute service. To John Merryman, thank you for being one of my closest friends. As I've long said, Master Choa was the inspiration, and you were the perspiration in organizing and writing down the teachings. Stephen and I have endless gratitude for all of the work you've put into this. I could not have written this book without the unfailing love and support of my wife, Linda, and my son, Jonah. I always tell you how thankful I am to be able to share life's journey with you both. Linda, you are so loving and warm and nurturing to everyone. Jonah, I couldn't be prouder of the man you are becoming. A thanks goes out to my parents for the wonderful job they did raising me, to my sister Elisa Pacht who is a fantastic person, wife, and mother; and to my dearly departed sister Leslie Ayn, who inspired me on this healing path more than she could have ever known.

I've been blessed with a number of great teachers in the mind-body healing field. Principal among these have been Gay Hendricks, Matt Sison, Cal Banyan, Tad James, Dr. Richard Bartlett, Paul Wong, Gary Craig, Bill Harris, Frank Kinslow, and Michael Langford. Thank you all for being part of my life and for helping me to evolve. And of course, many thanks to Jennifer and Haven at Sounds True; we're proud to be part of your author roster.

ERIC B. ROBINS, MD

This book would not have been possible without the contributions of many, many people. And here are just a few to whom I am indebted: first, of course, to Grandmaster Choa Kok Sui, for his amazingly clear and precise teachings on complex spiritual topics, without which there simply would have been no book. His teachings gave me a "spiritual home." To Master Stephen Co and Eric Robins, for their friendship and partnership. To my wife, Betsy, and son, David, for their boundless support and patience, and for enduring—once again—my many long hours in the office while forgoing Little League games and other family gatherings. I love them and owe them greatly. To my parents, who, though they remain a little unsure about the nature of the topics I've chosen to write about, are nonetheless proud of the final product. To the great team at Sounds True, especially Haven Iverson, for her deft stewardship of the manuscript, and Jennifer Brown, for "bringing us into the fold." To all the truly outstanding individuals in Pranic Healing who offered ideas, stories, testimonials, and their experiences of these exercises and other aspects of Grandmaster Choa's teachings.

JOHN MERRYMAN

Introduction   Why Do So Many People Have Low Energy?

People grumble about it constantly. Physicians hear it more than any other complaint. We now even have a variety of very popular drinks to remedy it.

"It" is fatigue, sluggishness, low energy.

In a contemporary world where we have an abundance of conveniences and automation available to us, it seems we have much less of the two things that modern technology was supposed to give us more of: time and energy. Time management is a subject beyond my expertise (and I struggle with it at times myself), but I have spent a substantial portion of my career as a physician studying the topic of energy—and more specifically, the question: why do people have low energy?

Let me begin by addressing the root of the problem of low energy: our lack of understanding regarding the true nature of our energy, or what other cultures call our life force, *chi* (in China), or *prana* (in India).

It's unfortunate that my own profession, Western medical science, has been perhaps the biggest stumbling block to a fuller comprehension of this life force. During my four years of medical school and six years of residency—and it wasn't that long ago—we were taught next to nothing about the body's energy. If a patient came in complaining of fatigue or low energy, we were instructed to take a full medical history and to run a number of tests to see if we could diagnose a medical cause for it, such as anemia, diabetes, hypothyroidism, sleep apnea, and so on. Of course, it is important to run such tests to rule out serious health problems, but every physician will tell you that, more often than not, such tests reveal nothing. All we can do in these cases is simply tell the patients that there is nothing medically wrong with them, though some physicians will go so far as to tell someone the problem "is in your head," or it's "just stress," which is just a convenient way to blame the patient for an illness that the physician can't fully explain or "fix." Patients often leave such an encounter feeling some sense of relief because they now know nothing serious is wrong, but they also go home largely unsatisfied, mainly because they're going home still tired, still fatigued, still depleted. What they don't realize is that Western medical science has no treatment to help people "get more energy."

It's because of such encounters, as well as the growing understanding—by the public and by enlightened physicians—of the limits of allopathic, or Western, medicine, that alternative medical treatments have become increasingly popular over the last several decades. And what is the major philosophical tenet underpinning most alternative medicine? It's the belief that the body's energy is not simply some theoretical concept or a verbal metaphor for physical prowess, but a real, tangible force.

Let me expand on this fundamental principle and offer what I see as the essential beliefs of alternative medicine, for these beliefs are also the basis for the energy-boosting routine you will read about in this book:

1. **The body heals itself.** Your body has a marvelous innate ability to heal. Medical interventions simply help this natural process. Diagnostic tests can give us a more accurate picture of a particular ailment. Antibiotics can give your natural immune system a helping hand. Surgery can correct a traumatic injury. But only the body itself can perform actual healing.

2. **Some sort of energy flows through the body to facilitate this healing.** Your body has an energy system, the same way it has a circulatory system, a musculoskeletal system, a nervous system, an endocrine system, and so on. The energy system of your body surrounds and interpenetrates your physical structures, and it is through this energy system that healing energy flows.

3. **The nature of this energy is to flow.** When the energy is flowing smoothly and plentifully, a state of physical and emotional health exists. When the smooth flow of this energy is interrupted—through either a depletion of the energy or a blockage in the system—the body becomes unbalanced, and the result is low energy. If this

energetic imbalance continues and the energy remains low for a period of time, this can lead to physical and emotional, or stress-related, ailments.

4. **This energy is quantifiable and measurable—if only by the way you feel.** And "how you feel" is a perfectly legitimate and accurate measurement of your health and energy. One of the most basic questions you can ask yourself regarding your health is this: do I have all the energy I want and need to live the life I want? If you answer no, then you can probably consider yourself as having low energy.

5. **Maintenance of this energetic equilibrium is essential for proper health, vitality, and energy.** In order to be healthy and to feel good—to have all the energy you want—your energy system must be in a state of homeostasis, which is, according to the dictionary, "a relatively stable state of equilibrium between the different but interdependent elements of an organism." This simply means your energy must be in a constant state of dynamic flow: not too much or too little in any area and always moving at a steady pace throughout your body without interruption or impediment.

6. **This energy can be cultivated, controlled, and increased—with the right methods and proper training.** Perhaps this is the most important point of all. With some alternative healing modalities, this energy is increased by someone acting upon you—for example, an acupuncturist inserting needles into a certain part of the body to unblock or facilitate the flow of chi or a Reiki practitioner directing energy into the body. In others, such as yoga or *chi kung,* you learn techniques to increase the energy yourself.

We wrote this book to give you the right methods and proper training you will need to balance and build your energy. If you don't believe you have all the energy you want or need to live the life you want—if you feel worn out, or just feel you look worn out—this book will help you.

* * *

Let's now discuss the reasons people have low energy. If we exclude illness or pathology—diagnostically verifiable diseases or medical conditions such as diabetes, cancer, and autoimmune disorders, many of which obviously can reduce your energy—there are, in my view, three main reasons people have chronically low energy: heredity, personal choices, and life situations and emotional reactions to them. I'll touch only briefly on the first two because they're fairly obvious, but I want to spend more time on the third, the emotional factor, because it is the most important and also the least understood.

The first factor that influences our flow and level of energy is heredity. It stands to reason that if we have an energy system the same way we have a circulatory system or a nervous system, some people will have a stronger or more effective energy system than others. Some people will simply be born with more energy, the way some people are born with a better physique or better eyesight. This doesn't mean, however, that low energy can't be overcome. You can be born with a heart murmur or even one kidney and still lead a normal or very full life. It's the same with your energy level. You just need to have access to the the right methods and proper training to increase your energy.

The second factor causing low energy is personal choice, and this is a factor that can be controlled. Is there anyone today who doesn't believe that smoking or excess drinking can negatively affect their health and energy? Proper diet, nutrition, and exercise are also vital to well-being, and any personal regimen designed to increase energy should take these elements into account. In fact, it should begin with them—even before seeking out an "energy routine." If you eat poorly, get no exercise, and smoke a lot, don't expect this book to give you the secret to better health and more energy with no effort on your part. That's like being overweight, eating a high-fat, high-sodium diet, and expecting a physician to control your high blood pressure and high cholesterol with medication. It won't work.

I firmly believe that the third factor, our life situations and how we react to them emotionally, holds the key to understanding our entire energy system. In fact, I believe that most cases of stress-related health problems and low energy are attributable to how we process our emotions—and particularly our negative emotions. We all know the main stressors of modern life—career, relationships, children, financial pressures, and so on—and what they can do to us. A demanding job can drain your energy, leaving you with little for your family or yourself. A marriage or relationship and children can be a source of enormous comfort and joy, but they can also at times cause heartbreak, strain, and stress. Financial worries can cause sleepless nights, anxiety, and worry. All of these situations—or more accurately, *how you react emotionally to these situations*—have the potential to cause a stress reaction in the body, which triggers chemical and energetic changes that can significantly reduce your level of energy. Let me explain how this works. First and foremost, we need to understand that stress reactions and negative emotions aren't "in your head," as some physicians tell us; *they actually are in your body*. Here's how this happens. As mentioned earlier, you have not only a physical body but also an energy body. This energy body can be called your *aura*. An aura is composed of several interlocking energy fields, plus your energy centers, or *chakras*, and energy channels, or *meridians*. Together, these pieces make up your *energetic anatomy*, a term we will use frequently throughout the book. Your aura surrounds and interpenetrates your physical body, and it is in this aura that you hold all your emotions—positive and negative. The reason is simple: all emotions themselves are energy. Thus, whatever is in your energy field, or aura, whether it's good or bad, positive or negative, helpful or hurtful, is also in your physical body.

There are three general categories of harmful emotional energy that can cause physical problems: negative emotions, limiting beliefs, and traumatic memories. The most common negative emotions are anger and fear, and they're usually directed at ourselves, a person currently or formerly in our lives, or the general circumstances of our lives. (Of course, emotions such as anger and fear can play a constructive role in our health—there's nothing wrong with being fearful in a potentially dangerous situation, and many psychologists would say that becoming angry in reaction to an instance of injustice would be normal and healthy. But in general, negative emotions have a harmful effect on our energy supply and health.) Limiting beliefs are attitudes that we adopt during our formative years as a result of the behavior of an authority figure or our experience in the world. Limiting beliefs are almost always false, yet we act and live our lives as if they were true. For example, you may have always felt that you just weren't attractive enough or smart enough—despite evidence to the contrary. A traumatic memory is an unshakable or repeating image or recollection of a disturbing incident—for example, witnessing a terrible accident as a child or the death of a loved one.

In the energy body, these harmful emotional energies create "ripples" that become impediments to the smooth and balanced flow of prana throughout your aura. Think of these blockages as a kink in a garden hose. The area above the kink is congested; water pressure builds up. The area below the kink is depleted; water pressure decreases. It works the same way with your energy body. Negative emotions, limiting beliefs, and traumatic memories create little "dams" that interrupt the smooth flow of prana. Thus, some areas of your aura become congested, and others become depleted, but the result is that the entire energy body becomes unbalanced. And as a result, health problems can arise in the parts of your physical body where you are holding these harmful emotional energies.

Here's a very important point to understand about destructive emotional energies in the body: there is *always* a physical feeling underlying any negative emotion, limiting belief, or traumatic memory. Consider, for example, the emotion of sadness. Think about the last time you were sad to the point of actually being depressed. Notice that it wasn't just a thought, but a *feeling in your body*. People don't say, "I think sad." They say, "I *feel* sad." The muscles feel limp, the body feels heavy, and the posture often reflects the sadness and depression: shoulders slumped, head down, eyes averted. Think about the last time you were anxious or fearful. More than likely, you felt it somewhere in your body. Perhaps it was your gastrointestinal system. If so, you may have thought to yourself, "Wow, my stomach is really in a knot," and that was quite likely physiologically true. Your stomach and/or intestines probably were tightly contracted in a spasm. It's also possible that your anxiety or fear contributed to constipation or diarrhea.

It works similarly with limiting beliefs. Perhaps your parents or a teacher told you repeatedly that you'd never amount to anything, and, as a result, you grew up with a lack of confidence and a poor self-image. This sort of conditioning could manifest as any number of unproductive attitudes and behaviors in adulthood, but one might be the belief that you're not smart enough to make good decisions. So you become indecisive or overly cautious because you're terrified of making a mistake or the wrong decision. And physically, each time you have to make a choice of some consequence, your neck muscles tense or your jaw clenches or your chest gets tight and it's difficult to breathe. And that's just one example of the physical feelings limiting beliefs might produce.

In my experience as a physician, traumatic memories are almost *always* held tightly somewhere in the physical body. Whenever patients tell me about a traumatic memory from their past, the first question I ask is, "When you think about that event, where do you feel it in your body?" About 80 percent of the time or more, patients are able to tell me exactly where they feel the emotional memory—as pain or discomfort—in their bodies.

It's important to note that, when dealing with all these harmful negative energies stuck in the body, quite often the physical feelings they generate are triggered so quickly and automatically that many people don't make a cause-and-effect connection between a feeling of depression or a traumatic memory and fatigue or physical discomfort unless it is brought to their attention in therapy or through some cognitive self-awareness technique. The indecisive adult in the limiting belief example mentioned earlier may not be aware of why or how his jaw gets so tense when he has to make a decision. Or, as is the case with the roughly 20 percent of women who say they were sexually abused but are unable to locate an emotional pain in their bodies, it's not that the memory is *not* held in their bodies, it's just that the women are so dissociated from their bodies, or they have buried the incident so completely, that they can't identify the feeling, let alone the location of the feeling.

In all these cases, the physical feelings are there; it's just that many times, we aren't sufficiently tuned into our bodies to feel them. And for good reason: when we're young we're taught to hold in our thoughts and feelings about difficult or painful experiences; we're told that it's not okay to feel or express emotions such as anger or anxiety. In fact, we're not even supposed to talk about them, especially if they're negative or uncomfortable—for us or for others. The problem with this is obvious: life is going to provoke anger or anxiety responses; it's inevitable. Suppressing these feelings—either because of conditioning or the quite natural fear of the pain and discomfort that would arise should we acknowledge them consciously—takes a tremendous amount of our energy and attention. Even if we're not always aware of our efforts, many of us work very hard to prevent ourselves from feeling our emotions. It's exhausting work, and this ongoing effort to bottle them up and keep them from conscious awareness is a prime source of not only general fatigue but also physical maladies.

For instance, it's fairly common to store negative feelings as unconscious contractions of the smooth muscles or skeletal muscles. The smooth muscles are those muscles functioning automatically in our body, without our conscious control, such as the musculature of the stomach, the bladder, the blood vessels, and the air passages. Holding unresolved emotions in the smooth muscles for a prolonged period can produce health problems such as irritable bowel syndrome, migraine headaches, high blood pressure, and asthma. The skeletal muscles are those muscles that we do have conscious control over, such as those involved with our arms and legs, the joints of movement, our facial expressions, and so on.

If you hold a suppressed traumatic memory in the skeletal muscles, it may present itself as chronic pain in your neck, shoulders, or back. Or you may be plagued by frequent tension headaches, temporomandibular joint (TMJ) disorder, or fibromyalgia.

These sorts of common maladies are marked by two characteristics: first, their cause is undetectable through modern medical scientific testing; and second, the symptoms are real enough—and often debilitating. Thus, because the functioning of the body is impaired in some unknown way, physicians call such conditions "functional ailments," and they account for a significant number of visits to the physician. Doctors may attribute the cause to stress, and they will usually only treat the physical symptoms—almost always with medication (inhalers for asthma, antispasmodics for irritable bowel syndrome, muscle relaxers for tight muscles, and so on). This is because they *can't* treat the cause—since the cause is energetic and emotional, not physiological. My hope is that some day, through the growing understanding of our life force and energy medicine, physicians will be able to write on a patient's chart a diagnosis of "energetic blockage due to unresolved emotional trauma" and prescribe an appropriate energetic or emotional treatment.

ERIC B. ROBINS, MD

HOW TO USE THIS BOOK

Here's a brief guide on how this book is organized so that you may get the most from it. It would certainly be best for your intellectual understanding of the body's energy system and how it works if you read the book in proper chapter-by-chapter sequence, but if you want a quick read and wish to get right to the exercises, you can go directly to chapter 6, "Performing the Nine Energizing Breaths." The exercises will still work for you and produce the energy you want even if you don't have a full understanding of your energetic anatomy, though we would still caution you to follow carefully all the directions and admonitions in that chapter.

If you read the book chapter by chapter, you'll find the philosophical and practical underpinnings of the Nine Energizing Breaths in Parts One and Two, followed by the exercise routine itself in Part Three, a variety of complementary meditations and supplemental energy exercises in Part Four, and finally, some appendices for those interested in additional material.

Part One is entitled "A Spiritual and Energetic Framework for the Contemporary World," and it details how Grandmaster Choa Kok Sui developed and introduced to the world Pranic Healing, his exhaustively detailed energy healing system, and Arhatic Yoga, his synthesis of various yoga and spiritual traditions. This discussion provides perspective and context for the Nine Energizing Breaths, as it also shows how these exercises fit into the larger background of his teachings.

Part Two, entitled "Building Your Energetic Foundation," begins with chapter 2, and here we go into more depth about prana, the universal life force that our body uses to power all its tasks, and our energetic anatomy, or our personal energy field, also known as the aura. Part Two also contains a summary of the key elements that characterize truly effective energy-generating practices and how the Nine Energizing Breaths utilize these elements for optimal personal energy production and health.

Proper pranic breathing is covered in chapter 3. Pranic breathing is controlled abdominal breathing performed with the right rhythm (so many beats per inhalation and exhalation) and retention (a critical pause between inhalation and exhalation). The Nine Energizing Breaths are powered by correct pranic breathing, in addition to body postures and "locks," which are muscular contractions in a certain part of the body that build up and/or direct the prana in a specific way, so attention to performing the breath with accuracy can't be emphasized enough.

Chapter 4 addresses Energetic Hygiene, which is a bonus from Grandmaster Choa's more advanced teachings. Energetic Hygiene is a set of rules and practices that keep your personal energy tank clean and full. It is a large topic, and there are many Energetic Hygiene techniques. However, we provide in this book three of the simplest and most effective methods for the care and maintenance of your energetic system: dietary recommendations, cutting the "energetic cords" that often drain your energy, and saltwater baths. These techniques are remarkably effective for increasing your stamina, and they are an excellent complement to the Nine Energizing Breaths.

Chapter 5 contains instruction in the Cleansing Physical Exercises referenced earlier. This set of mild twists and stretches is easy to perform, requiring little strength and flexibility, yet its ability to boost your energy by helping you expel dirty prana is amazing. The exercises make a good warm-up for the Nine Energizing Breaths.

Part Three, "The Nine Energizing Breaths," is the centerpiece of the book, and it takes you step-by-step through the routine as it should be practiced daily. It also includes a discussion of these energy-generating exercises in general, as well as the history of the Nine Energizing Breaths and why they increase your energy and support longevity and youthfulness.

Part Four, entitled "Advanced Practices for Enhanced Purification and Sustained Energy," includes several chapters with routines that you can add as a complement to the Nine Energizing Breaths. If you can make time for them in your daily practice, they will definitely accelerate your personal energy development. They include three simple but powerful meditations and feature Meditation on Twin Hearts, the foundational meditation of Grandmaster Choa's teachings. The supplemental energy exercises include the Tiger Breath and Five Points Energy Distribution, both of which will give you an extra boost, plus add some variety to your practice. This part concludes with some advice on helping you construct a daily practice regimen.

At the end of the book, there are three appendices, the first of which, appendix A, explains a topic from Pranic Healing called the Seven Healing Factors. These are rules that help determine how effective any healing effort—traditional, alternative, or energetic—will be. However, since practicing exercises that boost your own vitality and energy is nothing if not *self*-healing, reading about the Seven Healing Factors should enhance your understanding and practice of the Nine Energizing Breaths. Appendix B includes a brief summary of the major principles of three of the most popular energy practices: yoga, chi kung, and *tai chi chuan*. These three modalities are referenced frequently in the book because the Nine Energizing Breaths share many characteristic with them. In fact, the Nine Energizing Breaths may be said to be a distillation of the best of these practices. Finally, appendix C is a resource section in which we list and describe the various Pranic Healing and Arhatic Yoga classes offered throughout the world.

We will frequently discuss topics from both the physiological and the energetic perspective. That is, we will talk about a particular situation or exercise in terms of how it affects not only your physical anatomy (that is, the musculoskeletal and biochemical impact) but also your energetic anatomy. It's important that you understand the "energetic truth" behind many of the things you do and how your actions positively and negatively affect your overall level of energy.

It is our fondest wish that you use the power of prana to supercharge your energy, revitalize your health, and rejuvenate your body. Whether you feel like your "tank" is always drained, or you find yourself dragging yourself from home to work and back again each day, or you're just always too tired to get involved with activities you'd like to do, this book has an answer for you. The Nine Energizing Breaths and the related exercises can open the door for you to a healthier, more energized body and an invigorated life.

Part One

A Spiritual and Energetic Framework

for the Contemporary World

Chapter 1   "You Can't Serve on an Empty Stomach"

Pranic healer Wendy Scott used to have to drive regularly from Los Angeles to Oregon and back for family and business reasons. It was a tedious and mind-numbing 900-mile trip. To stay awake and alert, however, she didn't rely on Starbucks cappuccinos, caffeinated soft drinks, or even the many popular energy drinks; she used the Nine Energizing Breaths. "I would pull over at rest stops and just do the routine," she says. "Other people would be standing there smoking cigarettes and drinking coffee. I got some strange looks, but after doing the exercises, my body would be physically strengthened, I was more relaxed, and most important, I was more alert for the long drive."

During a question-and-answer session at an advanced meditation course a few years ago, Grandmaster Choa Kok Sui listened intently as a longtime student told him about his financial difficulties. The student was concerned that his erratic work history and meager income were impeding his pursuit of energy healing and spiritual studies, and he didn't know how to reconcile his basic material needs with his higher aspirations. Grandmaster Choa reflected for a moment, and then offered the student—who had had money problems for quite a while—a most unexpected response: "It may be time for you to take a break in your studies. Take a year or more off, until you get your finances stabilized. Then come back to healing and meditation. But get your finances in order first."

The class was very surprised. After all, this was a group of senior students; they were experienced healers and highly committed practitioners of

Arhatic Yoga, Grandmaster Choa's blend of yoga practices and various other select esoteric meditation techniques. And it's fair to say there were more than a few whose finances had suffered as they paid more attention to their highly intensive training with Grandmaster Choa than to making a living.

Yet, as Grandmaster Choa explained himself further, you could see the meaning of his lesson sink in. It's not like it was centuries ago, when villagers would support the local holy man or monk, he said. Begging for a living, as some monks did then, isn't much of a career path. You can't focus exclusively on learning esoteric teachings and ignore the need to have a regular income, he continued. Yes, in parts of the less-developed world there may yet be local communities that provide financial support for their spiritual leader. And there are still monasteries and cloistered orders where monks and nuns lead lives of self-imposed poverty while praying for humanity. But a life path of material austerity and spiritual focus has always been a choice made by very few people throughout history—and even fewer people in the modern world.

For serious students of Arhatic Yoga, many of whom hold high-minded ideals of using their meditation practices and healing ability in service to the world to make it a better place, Grandmaster Choa stressed, it's even more important to understand the need to have steady, reliable earnings.

He concluded his answer by saying, "You can't serve on an empty stomach."

Perhaps no anecdote better illustrates Grandmaster Choa's efforts to create a body of teachings that embraces both the subtlety of profound spiritual wisdom and the bedrock practicality of present-day life than his lesson that day: "You can't serve on an empty stomach."

It's also a perfect example of the philosophical context from which the Nine Energizing Breaths are drawn. Grandmaster Choa spent over two decades developing a system of thought, study, and practice that balances the needs of mind, body, and spirit:

- It promotes spiritual development but also emphasizes the importance of making a productive living.
- It expands the spiritual consciousness but also infuses the physical body with energy and strength.
- It urges its practitioners to reach upward for enlightenment but also to remain rooted on the earth to serve.

In short, it's a spiritual, healing, and energetic framework for the contemporary world.

All of Grandmaster Choa's teachings spring from that framework, including the Nine Energizing Breaths, so it would be helpful here at the outset to explain in a little more detail how Grandmaster Choa Kok Sui developed the many exercises, meditations, techniques, and practices of Pranic Healing and Arhatic Yoga. Learning the background of his system will give you greater insights into the Nine Energizing Breaths and how best to use them.

* * *

Grandmaster Choa Kok Sui was born in 1952 in the Philippines, attended Roman Catholic schools before receiving a degree in chemical engineering, and then went on to have a successful career as a businessman before turning full-time to researching, refining, and teaching his healing and spiritual systems. These include Pranic Healing, a simple but highly effective method of using life force for healing that has been described as "acupuncture without needles," and Arhatic Yoga, an eclectic synthesis of powerful meditations and energy-generating physical and breathing exercises. *Pranic* comes from *prana*, the Indian word for "life force." It is also known as *chi* in Chinese, *ki* in Japanese, *mana* throughout Polynesia, and *ruach* in ancient Hebrew. *Arhatic* derives from *arhat*, the Indian word for one who is "highly developed" or "highly evolved."

Grandmaster Choa became interested in paranormal and spiritual topics in his early teens, spending hours reading and practicing the teachings of the Rosicrucians, Theosophy, Astara, Huna, Kabbalah, and numerous similar systems. He had the good fortune to meet a number of highly proficient psychics, psychic healers, and clairvoyants (people with the ability to see the aura, or energy field, of animate objects) in the Philippines and worked with them almost daily throughout his twenties and early thirties. His primary focus initially was energy healing, and he began by researching a variety of such systems, including Chinese medical chi kung, Therapeutic Touch, Reiki, unguided "energy healing" (energy healing conducted by an untrained person who simply has the "gift" of healing), and many others. His research revealed that, while all these various healing systems were effective in certain circumstances and with the proper experienced healer, they also had limitations that he wanted to overcome. For instance, in Chinese medical chi kung systems, you are taught exercises to increase your own chi and then use it on the patient, but you still end up running down your own battery in the course of treatment. Other modalities use the same basic treatment for every malady—usually transmitting energy into the patient in some way—but Grandmaster Choa's own experiments indicated that each health problem produces a unique disruption to the body's energy system, which suggested a more individualized treatment approach. And he found no one system that really had the sort of precision or step-by-step approach he thought was needed. As he wrote, "Healing at that time was more of an art rather than a science, because concepts, terminologies, principles, techniques and methodologies were non-existent or were not clear."[1] Noting also that most energy healing systems required extensive training and practice, he also wanted his techniques to be much easier to use. His ultimate goal was to develop a "very effective healing system which ordinary people can learn in just a short period of time."[2]

Thus, Grandmaster Choa established several clinics in the Philippines, employing both traditional medical practitioners and energy healers to work on people with a variety of health problems—from routine ailments such as sore throats and influenza to more complex and serious disorders such as congestive heart failure and cancer. Most important, he employed two of the most renowned clairvoyants in the Philippines independently of each other—in effect, using each to cross-check the observations of the other—to ensure a degree of rigor in his studies. These clairvoyants would observe the specific disruptions that each illness or physical problem brings about in the body's energy field. Grandmaster Choa then used their readings of the aura to design a precise sequence of steps to reverse those negative energy changes and bring about healing for each particular health problem.

During this same period, from the 1970s through the early 1980s, he also experimented exhaustively with a variety of meditations and energy-generating techniques from such spiritual traditions as Taoism, Buddhism, Hinduism, Zoroastrianism, and Sufism, among many others. He also studied and practiced a variety of different types of yoga, including *raja* yoga, *karma* yoga, *laya* or *kundalini* yoga, *gnana* yoga, *bhakti* yoga, *mantra* yoga, and *hatha* yoga. As he progressed deeper into his esoteric studies, Grandmaster Choa began receiving instruction from Mahaguruji Mei Ling, also known as the renowned Tibetan Buddhist Bodhisattva Padmasambhava, who then became Grandmaster Choa's spiritual teacher. This advanced guidance accelerated his study exponentially, and he began having the same clairvoyants who helped him document the efficacy of energy healing modalities observe him while he practiced various high-level meditations.

Just as he did with Pranic Healing, Grandmaster Choa then recorded their readings on the changes in his aura each different technique produced. His goal was to create a logical, sequential system for spiritual development that could be learned and practiced by the "average person"—that is, someone who wants to progress spiritually but has no desire to retreat from modern society to a mountaintop or leave behind career, current relationships, or other worldly commitments.

In the early and mid-1980s, in preparation for going public with his work and beginning to teach, Grandmaster Choa began to pull together and more formally document his findings. The result was a comprehensive yet simple-to-learn multilevel system of energy healing, Pranic Healing, and spiritual development, Arhatic Yoga.

The principles that underlie both Pranic Healing and Arhatic Yoga include many familiar terms, but it will be instructive to present these terms here at the beginning because different esoteric philosophies and religious teachings often have slightly different interpretations of them.

As mentioned earlier, prana is the term for the universal life force that powers everything we do. Modern English doesn't really have a single equivalent word for this life force, but many Eastern and ancient languages have long referred to it. Prana is also called "subtle energy."

The aura is your personal energy field, but you don't have just a single aura. Rather, the aura is a set of several interlocking energy fields that surround and interpenetrate the physical body. Each person has three auras: the inner aura, an "inner shield" of prana that stretches out about six inches from the physical body (if the person is healthy); the outer aura, an "exterior casing" of prana that envelops both the physical body and the inner aura and that can reach out to many feet beyond the physical body; and the health aura, which is a series of two foot-long pranic beams that emanate from the body's pores like long tendrils and extend well into the outer aura.

Your aura, or energy field, contains chakras and meridians. *Chakra*, which comes from the Sanskrit word for "wheel," is a term for the body's energy transformers that take in and distribute life force throughout the energy body via the meridians. You have eleven major chakras and many minor chakras. Each chakra controls and directs energy to one or more organs. The meridians are the energy channels, or "energy highways," of your aura. The meridians take energy from the chakras and carry it throughout the body. The meridians correspond to acupuncture energy channels, and also to *nadi* in yogic literature.

Together, this three-dimensional arrangement of auras, chakras, and meridians that surround and interpenetrate the physical body comprises what is called your energetic anatomy, or energy body.

Along with this energetic anatomy, each of us has a two-part Soul that includes the Higher Soul, which is the near-God presence that goes by a variety of names in different spiritual systems, including the Atma and the Higher Buddha Nature, as well as the Incarnated Soul, a portion of the Higher Soul that is extended downward and "ensouled" in the physical body shortly before birth. When yogis speak of "soul realization," they are referring to a connection with the Higher Soul. At the top of the energy body, extending upward from the crown chakra at the top of our head, is the spiritual cord, which appears to clairvoyant observation as a multicolored rainbow strand that connects the Incarnated Soul to the Higher Soul. Further up above the Higher Soul, this spiritual cord also connects the Higher Soul to the Divine Spark, which is the highest aspect of God that we can comprehend in this plane. The second union of yoga, or God realization, is union with the Divine Spark.

In both Pranic Healing and Arhatic Yoga, students learn pranic breathing, which is deep abdominal breathing performed with a certain rhythm—so many counts on the inhalation and so many on the exhalation. These special rhythms maximize the amount of prana generated, which can then be used for healing others, self-healing, or self-energizing. Pranic breathing is also used during meditation.

There are also some terms particular to Pranic Healing that will be beneficial for you to know. The first of these is scanning, which refers to the ability to feel the subtle energy of the aura around all living things. Scanning is first taught in Basic Pranic Healing and involves hand sensitization, which is learning to open up the palm chakras, located in the center of the hands, to enable students to feel energetic changes in the aura during healing or during class experiments. Scanning allows healers to detect areas of the aura or specific chakras that are out of balance—either because of congestion (too much dirty energy) or depletion (energetic insufficiency). Sweeping, or cleaning, refers to using simple hand movements to remove areas of energetic congestion or contamination so that fresh prana can move into the area to facilitate healing. Sweeping is carried out on the overall aura, a specific body part, or an individual chakra with long strokes or small circular movements. Energizing involves drawing in prana through one chakra and projecting it out through one or both palm chakras during a pranic healing treatment into a particular chakra or area of the aura. Energizing is always preceded by sweeping. Stabilizing refers to energizing a chakra or area of the aura with light-blue prana after healing to keep the fresh energy from leaking out. Light-blue prana has an inhibiting quality that makes it ideal for this purpose.

In Pranic Healing, two types of prana are used. The first is white prana— pale, bright, elemental healing energy—to remedy simple health problems. The second is colored prana—various shades of prana, each with different healing characteristics—which is used to address more complex or serious health problems. Colored prana creates a more focused effect on the energy field and the chakras. Here is a list of the types of colored prana and their qualities:

- **Red** Warm, expansive, dilating, stimulating, strengthening
- **Orange** Expelling, splitting, exploding, decongesting
- **Yellow** Stimulating, cementing, repairing
- **Green** Breaking down, disinfecting, dissolving
- **Blue** Disinfecting, localizing, stabilizing, cooling
- **Violet** Has properties of all pranas
- **Electric violet and gold** Highly refined pranas used for special purposes by experienced pranic healers

Electric violet prana appears to clairvoyant observation as lightning, and, like regular violet, it has the properties of all pranas. Gold prana is similar to electric violet prana but is less fluid and has a strong regenerative effect on the body.

There is also a unique prana called divine spiritual energy, which is the blindingly bright white prana that flows downward from the Higher Soul during certain meditations and that has the highest degree of refinement of all the pranas.

* * *

There is one other bit of background material that we want to cover here in chapter 1, and that is an examination of the four key traits of Grandmaster Choa's work. They've been suggested implicitly already, but we'd like to offer a few examples of how these characteristics are displayed across the range of his teachings before illustrating how they are embodied in the Nine Energizing Breaths. The first of these characteristics is simplicity.

One of Grandmaster Choa's primary goals was to make his teachings accessible to everyone, and to that end, his classes are filled with examples of complex topics made simple. In Kriyashakti, the class that teaches the "science of materialization," there are numerous step-by-step techniques that enable students to sharpen their focus on what they want, set their minds to that focus, and then meditate and take action in such a way as to bring about those results. In Pranic Feng Shui, Grandmaster Choa dispenses with most of the aspects of traditional Feng Shui, such as consideration of birth date, precise placement of objects, and selection of colors, as well as such inordinately complex techniques as laying the *bagua* diagram over a building to ensure proper energy flow. Instead, he focuses on a handful of form and direction changes for the home or workplace that, he demonstrates, account for over 80 percent of the positive Feng Shui that can be produced. These changes include, for instance, the optimum location for the front door of your home—the building's "energetic mouth"—and how to fix the Feng Shui of a front door that faces the wrong direction simply, without having to engage in an expensive remodel. (To get 100 percent perfect Feng Shui is almost impossible, according to Grandmaster Choa.)

But perhaps none of his classes provides as clear an example of simplicity as the "cookbook approach" to remedying physical and psychological ailments he developed in Pranic Healing. It works like this: after learning the fundamentals, such as pranic breathing, hand sensitization, scanning, and energizing—usually within the time frame of a two-day class—a student need only turn to the particular page in a Pranic Healing textbook for a specific ailment and follow the step-by-step instructions for everything from allergies to gallstones to varicose veins. Each health problem has a similarly specific, yet simple, step-by-step healing sequence.

"Pranic Healing was really easy to learn," says longtime student Karla Alvarez. "I had no previous experience with energy work, chakras, or healing of any kind before I took the first class. After the first day, we were told to go home and apply what we had learned, and I immediately applied the healing protocol on my mother, who at the time suffered from arthritis-like symptoms in the legs and lower back. The pain prevented her from sitting or lying comfortably and from driving without pain. I simply followed the step-by-step instructions, and amazingly she felt immediate relief of pain and stiffness. After that session she asked me to continue working on her, and after four months, all symptoms and pain disappeared! I was surprised to discover that although I was a beginner, I was still able to apply the technique and actually give quick relief to a loved one!"

The second hallmark of Grandmaster Choa's work is practicality. Grandmaster Choa was trained as a chemical engineer, so you often see in his teachings a degree of precision and specificity that is unusual in books and classes on alternative healing, energy work, or spirituality. And since he was also a successful businessman, his teachings place a high premium on "reality." Theory is fine to establish a context, but ultimately, all his teachings have to be efficient and work in the real world. That means his methods are logical, succinct, and results-oriented.

The earlier anecdote about his advice to the financially challenged student is just one example of his practicality. The origin of his program to feed the homeless provides another. About ten years ago, during one of his frequent teaching trips to the West Coast, Grandmaster Choa observed Los Angeles's large homeless population milling about. Moved by their plight, he instructed the students walking with him to go to a local McDonald's, purchase several large sacks of hamburgers, and distribute them to the homeless. Since Grandmaster Choa was, for the purposes of keeping his personal energy supply clean, a strict vegetarian, as were most of the students with him, this surprised many of them. However, as Grandmaster Choa explained, these weren't people concerned with healing or spirituality or an energetically clean diet. They were just trying to survive. "Their needs are very basic," he said. "Their bodies need simple nourishment, and they need to be given something they're likely to eat." Out of this experience came a worldwide program that provides food to the homeless and hungry.

Practicality is also evident in the sequence in which Grandmaster Choa developed his entire system. He began by asking, "What does humanity need? What would do the greatest good?" and proceeded with a series of the classes in a hierarchy of needs, focusing first on the physical body (much as he did with the hungry homeless in Los Angeles) by developing Basic Pranic Healing and Advanced Pranic Healing. Next, he developed a system for healing the emotions, Pranic Psychotherapy, followed by teachings to provide "financial healing" with Kriyashakti, his class on prosperity and manifestation. Only after those basic, more worldly needs were covered did he move on to more esoteric topics, such as spiritual development in Arhatic Yoga and then the even more advanced and specific classes, such as Pranic Feng Shui, Higher Clairvoyance, Sexual Alchemy, and others. More recently, he created perhaps the ultimate merger of spirituality and practicality with his course entitled Pranic Business Management, a class that applies his spiritual concepts to individual careers, entrepreneurship, and both small and large corporations.

Los Angeles television anchor and reporter Jennifer Sabih applied Pranic Feng Shui to her newsroom office and got immediate practical results. "My colleagues rolled their eyes when I came to work one day, pulled out a compass, then promptly swiveled my chair away from the 'nice' view and toward an unattractive wall," she says. "I couldn't blame them for laughing when I explained that according to Pranic Feng Shui, the energy from this direction would activate my basic chakra, allowing me to work longer and harder and think more effectively. But I suffered the snickers, because a few days later, it became clear to me how much more creatively and quickly I was writing my stories; the words seemed to just flow effortlessly. And I wasn't the only one who noticed a difference in the quality of my work. When we moved to a new studio, the news director told a manager making the seating plan to 'make sure Sabih's desk faces the right direction.' I thought at the time she was indulging me, but then a few days later, she confided to me that she had an important meeting coming up with her boss and quietly asked which direction her chair should face to maximize her negotiating power."

The third characteristic of Grandmaster Choa's work is perhaps the most unique, for it is an open challenge to anyone who is unsure of whether these teachings will work for them or not, and that is his focus on proof and not taking any teachings—including his own—for granted. The fact that he was working in a field that didn't lend itself easily to objective proof didn't discourage Grandmaster Choa; in fact, it only increased his resolve to develop a method to test his theories—thus, his great reliance on clairvoyant observation and scanning. Even his students get to find out for themselves just how well the techniques work, primarily through learning to scan. Scanning sounds a bit exotic, but we've all got the innate ability to feel subtle energy; it just needs to be "relearned and reactivated." Most students learn it in their first Basic Pranic Healing class, and those who do not usually pick it up with a couple weeks of practice.

Los Angeles resident Edward Andonian's initial experience with scanning was as the recipient of a Pranic Healing session that was so quick and subtle, yet powerful, that the visit still resonates with him eight years later. "I made an appointment to see a hypnotist to deal with some ongoing health and stress issues," he says. "I had thyroid problems and a very stressful work situation. The day I went to see her, I was feeling tremendous pressure in my chest. Before we did the hypnosis, she asked if she could do something first and began to move her hands in and out all around my body. I had no idea what she was doing, but within ninety seconds, I felt myself just melt. It was as if the entire weight of the day had been lifted from my body. The tension in my chest was completely gone. And this was *before* the hypnosis session. 'What did you do?!' I asked. 'Pranic Healing,' she replied. 'I scanned your aura to feel for energy imbalances and then fixed them.' I'll never forget the way she just waved her hands over me and just made the stress go away. It changed my life."

While scanning is important for healers to learn, it is also used to test the theories and assertions in Grandmaster Choa's other classes. For instance, in Pranic Feng Shui, when students are told that facing a certain direction while conducting business or negotiations will increase the likelihood of prosperity or success, they perform scanning exercises while facing that direction. They then repeat the experiment while facing other directions to compare and verify their original findings. Arhatic Yoga students often use mantras, which are certain sounds or words that, when repeated either aloud or silently, have a transformative effect on the mind or aura, when they meditate. So, for instance, when students are given a mantra that is supposed to increase the size of their spiritual cord, they scan the cord before and after using the mantra to see if the words have indeed increased the size of the spiritual cord.

Perhaps the best way to sum up Grandmaster Choa's emphasis on proof is with a line he repeated frequently in every class: "Don't take my word for it. Do the exercises and draw your own conclusions."

It may just be a personality trait of the sort of person drawn to energy work or people's reaction to the great scope of Grandmaster Choa's teachings when they're initially exposed to them, but it's not unusual for beginning and even advanced students to get a bit carried away and overload their lives with meditations, exercises, practice, classes, and so on—often to the exclusion of more worldly or practical considerations. Thus, the fourth characteristic of Grandmaster Choa's work is the notion of moderation, both in terms of the amount of time and energy devoted to practice and the expectations each person should have with regard to the speed of their progress.

Grandmaster Choa was very much against fanaticism in any form, and particularly spiritual fanaticism. Thus, in Arhatic Yoga, students are given a recommended schedule of meditations and other practices with sufficient flexibility that takes into account the other important aspects of their lives, such as work and family obligations, as well as recreation, vacation, and entertainment. Grandmaster Choa himself led a modest but certainly not ascetic life. He had an ashram in India to which he would retreat for spiritual rejuvenation and for high-level classes, but he also enjoyed traveling and was very fond of movies and restaurants. He had a wide range of interests and could strike up a conversation about world or local politics or business at a moment's notice. Grandmaster Choa was the very embodiment of the Buddha's Middle Path between worldly pleasure and self-denial, between spirituality and materialism.

His approach to moderation was found in his classes as well. In the Kriyashakti class on prosperity, for instance, students are given an ideal ratio to shoot for in their personal financial management: a certain amount for savings and a certain amount for tithing, but also a certain amount of disposable income for entertainment. And his Pranic Business Management course is filled with similar examples of moderation, such as specially developed meditations to cultivate better day-to-day decision-making skills.

But Grandmaster Choa also tried to instill moderation as a value in his students because to try to go too fast and get too far ahead of the teacher isn't always wise. At times, it can even be dangerous. Higher-level meditations produce a lot of energy that can create discomfort for people not used to having such refined and powerful prana in their own aura. Also, the Arhatic Yoga meditations, like many advanced yoga practices, are designed to awaken the kundalini, which is the powerful primordial force that lies coiled at the base of the spine. There are many stories in yogic literature of students who went off on their own or who tried to advance too quickly or without sufficient guidance from their teacher and had the very unpleasant experience of "kundalini syndrome." This is the uncontrolled awakening of the kundalini, which has been known to produce severe anxiety, uncontrolled sexual urges, chronic insomnia, overheating of the physical body, and even madness and financial ruin.

Senior student and pranic healer Daniel O'Hara experienced a host of problems after he neglected the principle of moderation and began practicing an advanced meditation without the proper preparation or grounding. "I wanted to progress through the meditations as quickly as I could," he says. "I wanted to go 'up the ladder' rapidly to higher-level practices. As a long-time martial artist, I looked at it this way: if you're given the choice between learning a simple white-belt technique and a more complex, flashier black-belt technique, most people would want to learn the trickier black-belt technique. That's how I was. So, after practicing the basic preparatory-level Arhatic Yoga exercises for a year, I figured out how to do level two and decided to skip level one—even though it's recommended that students practice level one for at least a year or even two. As a result, I became the 'poster boy' for what could go wrong when you go too fast. I had challenges in every area of my life, personally and professionally: relationship, finances, and work. It began to be resolved when, on the advice of Grandmaster Choa, I cut back my practice and began performing only Meditation on Twin Hearts, one of the more introductory practices, and temporarily stopped the powerful Arhatic Yoga meditations. I learned a hard lesson about moderation."

* * *

So, how do the Nine Energizing Breaths fit into Grandmaster Choa's larger spiritual, healing, and energetic framework? How do they reflect these characteristics? And most important, how do they address the problem of low physical energy while helping those who are so inclined to further develop spiritually?

First, the Nine Energizing Breaths are exceptionally *simple*—in their design and as a routine to perform. Each exercise has been distilled to the least complicated yet most effective set of movements. And the key adjustments built into them—the physical movements and breathing changes that increase their power exponentially while keeping the entire set of exercises just ten minutes long—are extremely subtle and simple to perform. The Nine Energizing Breaths are much like Pranic Healing: designed to be learned and put to use quickly by anyone. Unlike other energy-development routines, such as many forms of yoga or chi kung, the Nine Energizing Breaths do not require any special strength, flexibility, dexterity, or athletic ability.

Second, the emphasis on *practicality* in the Nine Energizing Breaths can be seen in the modifications to the exercises made by Grandmaster Choa. As you read in the story about Laura Appelgren in the preface, there are two versions of this routine: the "original" exercises and the "modified" version, which is the one presented in this book. The original routine, popularized by Edwin Dingle's Mentalphysics organization, while undeniably effective, is also quite long: the practitioner must build up over a period of time the ability to perform the whole routine, which takes an hour. With an engineer's attention to efficiency, Grandmaster Choa drew upon his extensive knowledge of the body's energetic anatomy and made a few simple adjustments to the exercises. As a result, he reduced the time it takes to do them to ten minutes, while increasing their power dramatically. The modified version is safer, too, as it allows students to begin performing the whole routine right away.

Third, Grandmaster Choa extended the same rigorous proof criteria to the practice of the Nine Energizing Breaths as he did with all his other teachings. Students are taught the exercises right after lunch, the time of low energy for most people. They also learn to scan their auras before and after performing the Nine Energizing Breaths so that they have a clearer sense as to how the routine actually does increase the size of their aura and chakras. They are usually surveyed as to their energy level before and after practicing.

And fourth, even though the Nine Energizing Breaths are powerful and the whole routine can be performed right away, beginning students are given a progressive schedule for practice, a plan that follows the principle of *moderation*. It would be easy enough to suggest that students push ahead and do more repetitions of each exercise and add in other higher-level variations to speed up their progress even further. But this could also lead to discomfort for some, as not everyone's physical bodies and auras are used to handling this surcharge of energy. So, as with all Pranic Healing and Arhatic Yoga practices, the best approach to getting the most out of the Nine Energizing Breaths is to practice diligently but sensibly.

* * *

How do the Nine Energizing Breaths work so well? What exactly takes place in your aura as you perform them that increases your supply of prana, boosts your energy, and rejuvenates your body? This will be covered in much greater detail when you learn to perform the exercises in chapter 6, but put simply, Grandmaster Choa has created a "forced energy" system. By this, we mean that the energy produced by many of his meditations and techniques such as the Nine Energizing Breaths is strong enough to force open any blockages in the chakras or meridians the way a plumber's snake unclogs a drain. It will also help smooth out and balance the energy in the aura, filling in areas of depletion. Since, as explained earlier, blockages and depletions in the aura are evidence of both low energy and possible health problems, the Nine Energizing Breaths balance and heal the aura—and with it the physical body. The result is more energy and better health for you.

It's important to note, however, that the level of prana generated by the Nine Energizing Breaths—even with the moderate practice schedule recommended here—can occasionally make some people uncomfortable, particularly as it breaks through some of those energetic/emotional ripples in the aura. Students who have an unusual number of emotional issues, for instance, might experience a welling up of sadness, fear, or anxiety as they practice the Nine Energizing Breaths. Or they might have a sudden urge to cry. Others might feel a bit jittery, as if they had consumed too much caffeine. None of these feelings are dangerous, and they will pass quickly, but some people might consider them unpleasant. Thus, as a safeguard against negative side effects, the book also includes a variety of complementary practices that help ensure smooth absorption of the additional prana the Nine Energizing Breaths generate. These include the previously mentioned pranic breathing; several types of Energetic Hygiene, the practice of keeping your personal energy tank clean and full; and the Cleansing Physical Exercises, a set of simple twists and stretches that also help keep your energy body clean.

Grandmaster Choa Kok Sui was fond of this engineering analogy to help explain the energetic changes his exercises and meditations produce and the remedies that guard against discomfort: if you increase the voltage flowing through low-quality wire, the impurities and non-conductive elements in the metal of the wire create excess friction and heat, and the current flow is slowed down. It's not an efficient method of energy flow. However, in high-quality wire, which has fewer impurities and greater conductivity, you can increase the current easily without creating friction and heat. More electricity can move at a faster rate through high-quality wire. It's much more efficient. Some people's energy bodies are like low-quality wire. They have many "impurities"—energetic and emotional blockages, areas of depletion, and so on—that inhibit the smooth flow of energy. And when a higher voltage flows through their bodies—as it will when they begin practicing the Nine Energizing Breaths—they may experience "friction" and "heat," which are the feelings of discomfort as the new energy breaks through those energetic blockages as noted above. But pranic breathing, Energetic Hygiene, and the Cleansing Physical Exercises help increase the cleanliness of the energy body. They help your energy body become like high-quality wire through which greater quantities of energy can flow rapidly and easily without friction and heat.

One last important point before we move on to the specific details of performing the Nine Energizing Breaths and related practices: the Nine Energizing Breaths, like Pranic Healing, are multileveled in their application. By that we mean that people come to Pranic Healing with a wide variety of motivations. Some are just looking for treatment options for a physical problem that has so far resisted traditional medical remedies. Others are merely curious and come to learn a simple alternative healing method that they can apply for themselves and their families and loved ones whenever problems arise—from the common cold to insomnia to arthritis pain. Still other people are more "spiritually ambitious"; they use Pranic Healing as their point of entry into more advanced esoteric classes, Arhatic Yoga training, and a life of deeper spiritual study. All these are perfectly fine motivations, and the same reasoning applies here with the Nine Energizing Breaths. We wrote the book to help people with low energy, and if that's the reason you're here, we're confident you'll find a set of exercises that will help you feel better and have more "juice" to do the things you want to do. If you want a breathing and physical movement routine to complement some similar practice you're already engaged in, such as yoga, tai chi, or the like, you should find that, too. But if, as you read, you find yourself more spiritually adventurous and interested in pursuing additional studies, we think you'll find some exercises and some esoteric "nuggets" that may well spark your further explorations, as well.

As with all of Grandmaster Choa's teachings, the Nine Energizing Breaths is a multileveled routine for body, mind, and spirit. It's up to you to decide how far you'd like to take it.

Part Two

Building Your
Energetic Foundation

Chapter 2   Prana Power

On the day that Robynn Lim first became acquainted with the Nine Energizing Breaths, she was suffering from a lingering headache as well as shoulder pain. She learned the routine after lunch on the second day of a lengthy and intensive two-day Pranic Healing class. Day two is often the point in the classes when the exercises are taught, as it is an "energetic low point" for most people. And Robynn was no different: her energy was low, and she was a bit groggy. After completing the Nine Energizing Breaths one time, however, she reported that not only was she invigorated and energized, but both her ailments were completely relieved. She found the routine to be "simple and easy."

The energy that sustains and vitalizes life is all around us. It's in the air we breathe and the earth upon which we walk. We get it from the food we eat and from the sun under which we live our lives. We are literally swimming in an ocean of this universal life force that we refer to as prana. Fortunately, we have been blessed with a body that has the natural capacity to absorb this energy—from the air, the sun, the earth, and our food—and use it efficiently to power every task we perform: from mundane instinctive physical chores such as moving our arm to pick up the phone, to deliberate mental activities such as planning a daily to-do list, to incredibly complex automatic functions such as cell regeneration and healing.

But consider this: if it is true that this life force is all around us—and it is—why then aren't we always energized and healthy? If this prana is available to us at virtually every turn in our life, and we take it in automatically, why should we ever be tired or sick or unhealthy? If we have ready access to an inexhaustible supply of the fuel our bodies and minds need, why should we ever become mentally fatigued, stressed out, or physically run down?

There are two very basic reasons:

1. There are different levels of energy absorption capability, and most people never learn higher-level practices that enable them to draw in the large quantity of life force needed to get and stay sufficiently charged for life's many tasks.

2. This energy, while extremely powerful, is also delicate; it's easily diminished or contaminated by poor diet, bad lifestyle choices, and other factors such as unresolved negative emotions. As a result, most people never learn how to maintain the purity, or quality, of their life force.

QUANTITY: PRANA EXCHANGE AND ABSORPTION

When we breathe, we inhale oxygen and exhale carbon dioxide. This process is known as *respiration,* and it is a continuous exchange of these two gases between us and our environment. Similarly, there is *pranic respiration,* or a *prana exchange,* between us and the outer world to help us get the energy we need. We absorb fresh life force—from the sun, the earth, the air, and our food—and we expel dirty or used-up energy back into the environment. The body consumes prana constantly, just as it does oxygen. And, like oxygen, the prana needs to be constantly replenished. It's a continuous cycle. However, as noted above, there are different levels of this energy exchange. We all have the inherent ability to absorb the baseline amount of prana we need to sustain life, which might be described as a "subsistence level" of energy exchange. At this level, we draw in and expel energy *unconsciously* and *passively*—that is, without willful intent, thought, or technique. The vast majority of people function at this subsistence level—and even this level works marvelously well in helping us meet our basic needs. However, to increase your personal supply of energy, to boost the quantity of the prana you take in, you need to learn and practice more effective methods of prana absorption and exchange. This is best achieved by learning to change your energy exchange level from *unconscious* and *passive* to *conscious* and *active*—and when this happens, you have the ability to take in enough prana to not only survive, but to thrive and live a more vigorous, energetic life.

QUALITY: ENERGETIC HYGIENE

In a world in which each living thing is a part of a larger universal energy system, we are always able to tap into this bioenergetic "organism" to get fresh prana. But while this energy is plentiful, it is also subtle and easily contaminated. Thus, we need to continuously perform what is called Energetic Hygiene, or the practice of keeping your personal energy tank clean and full. Energetic Hygiene helps ensure that the quality of your energy is high.

To improve the quality of your energy supply, you need to be aware of the two types of energetic contamination: environmental and emotional. Environmental energetic contamination is simple to understand: if you live in an area that has significant air, ground, or water pollution, the energy supply in that area will be contaminated as well. So if you perform breathing exercises in a large, heavily industrialized, highly polluted urban area such as Mexico City, for instance, the energy you will draw in will be of lower quality—that is, it will be much more contaminated—than the energy you would draw in while performing breathing exercises on a Hawaiian beach with cool ocean breezes. It also stands to reason that food grown in an energetically dirty area will be more contaminated than food grown in an energetically clean area.

Emotional contamination has three aspects—self-contamination, contamination from others, and contamination from what might be called "life circumstances"—and they all spring from the energetic fact that negative emotions, such as fear and anger, actually inhibit or deplete your energy when they are not acknowledged and processed in a productive way. Clairvoyants, people who have the ability, either naturally or through special training, to see life force can observe a person's energy aura get smaller and cloudier when he or she gets angry. In Pranic Healing, after people learn to scan, they can feel the aura shrink or move in as a person thinks negative thoughts. Thus, when we repeatedly hold only negative thoughts or emotions, such as fear and anger, or when we have unresolved memories of trauma, or when we hold on to limiting beliefs, we contaminate our personal energy supply; it gets congested or depleted—or both. Similarly, we can become emotionally contaminated by the negativity of others. We all have experienced the unpleasantness of being around someone who is constantly angry, depressed, or unhappy. This unpleasantness, which may take the form of general discomfort, fatigue, irritability, or even some stronger physical feeling such as an upset stomach, is actually an energetic interaction between our aura and the other person's aura. Because we are sensitive beings and what surrounds us has an effect on us, another person's chronically negative state can contaminate our energy supply. Finally, we can also become contaminated through our reaction to daily life situations. A short deadline at work, a tough boss, money troubles, or a child's difficulty at school are all common situations people face every day. These circumstances often prompt stress, anxiety, fear, and anger, all of which can bring about changes in our aura (energetic congestion or depletion leading to an imbalanced or uneven flow of prana), as well as biochemical changes in the body (our fight-or-flight impulse that includes increased adrenaline production, accelerated heart rate, and so on). All these changes sap our energy.

So, given what we've just outlined for you—the great level of pollution in our world today and the many sources of environmental and emotional contamination that surround us—it may seem as if it would be impossible to keep yourself energetically clean. But take heart! One of the hallmarks of Grandmaster Choa's system is providing simple techniques to overcome the "energetic shortcomings" of our modern world. This book is full of them. As Grandmaster Choa often said of the ever-present contamination in the world, "You can't make all the world's roads smooth, so you wear shoes." We can't change the fundamental degree of contamination around us, so we adapt and learn techniques to neutralize the dirty energy as best we can.

YOUR ENERGETIC ANATOMY

The quantity and quality of your personal energy supply is contained in a system perfectly designed to accommodate it. For just as we have a physical anatomy that is comprised of skin, bones, organs, muscles, and so on, we also have an energetic anatomy,[1] which is the three-dimensional arrangement of auras, chakras, and meridians explained in chapter 1. See figure 2.1 for a detailed representation of the energetic anatomy.

The chakras are the key power centers of the energetic anatomy, and it's important for you to have a better understanding of the eleven major chakras and the organs and parts of the body they regulate (see figure 2.2 on page 36 and table 2.1 on pages 39–40). Beginning at the top of the head, there is the crown chakra. The crown chakra controls and energizes the brain and pineal gland. It is also one of the body's main entry points of prana, and energizing the crown chakra energizes the entire body. It's similar to pouring water into a funnel; as prana enters the body through the crown, it flows throughout the entire body. The crown chakra is also the entry point of especially high-vibration prana generated during powerful meditations, since it is the aura's center of divine love.

The forehead chakra is located at the center of the forehead, close to the hairline, and this chakra regulates the entire nervous system. Like the

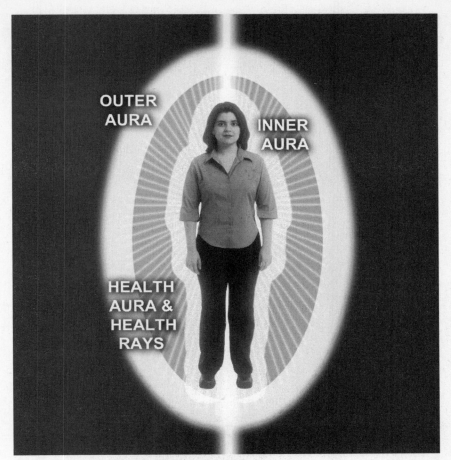

Figure 2.1 **The Auras of the Energetic Anatomy**

crown, it also energizes the pineal gland and can be used to direct prana throughout the rest of the body. The forehead chakra is the third eye, or spiritual eye, as it is known in some teachings. This is the chakra used for clairvoyance and higher consciousness perception and intuitive sensing.

The ajna chakra is located between the eyebrows and controls the pituitary gland and the entire body. The ajna chakra (or just the "ajna") is often called the *master chakra* because it governs the other chakras and also the endocrine system. The ajna is often mistakenly called the third eye, usually by adherents of a seven-chakra system. As noted above, the forehead chakra is the true third eye.

The throat chakra is located at the center of the throat. It controls and energizes the throat, and thyroid and parathyroid glands. It also has a correspondence with the sex chakra, as the throat chakra is the higher center

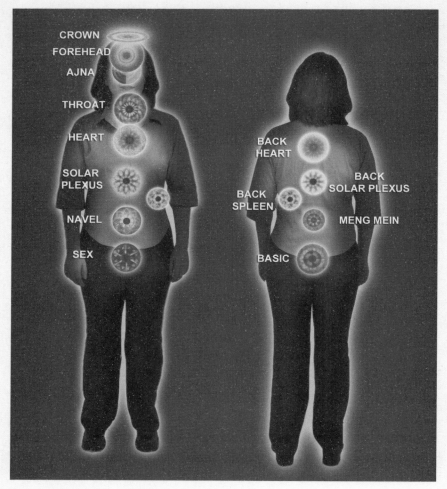

Figure 2.2 **The Eleven Major Chakras**

for creativity while the sex chakra is the lower center for creativity.

The heart chakra is located at the center of the chest and is one of several chakras with a front and back characteristic. The front heart chakra controls and energizes the heart and thymus gland, while the back heart chakra controls and energizes the heart and lungs. The heart chakra is important to many healing protocols because the thymus gland is so essential to the body's immune system. The heart chakra has a connection to both the solar plexus chakra and the crown chakra. Since it is the center of higher or refined emotions, the heart chakra is related to the solar plexus chakra, which is the center of lower emotions. And since it is the center of worldly love, it also relates to the crown, which is the center of divine love.

The solar plexus chakra is located in the depression just below the sternum and also has a front and back characteristic. It controls the key organs of digestion, including the stomach, liver, pancreas, and intestines. The solar plexus chakra is the seat of lower emotions, with the front solar plexus chakra governing expressed emotions (for example, fear that you let out as a loud cry) and the back solar plexus chakra governing suppressed emotions (for example, long-harbored resentments, unspoken feelings). Since there is so frequently an emotional component to many ailments, the solar plexus chakra is almost always included in Pranic Healing treatments.

The spleen chakra has two aspects, a front and a back. The front spleen chakra is located under the floating rib on the left side of the body, while the back spleen chakra is located directly behind the front spleen chakra. The spleen chakra is a crucial energy center, as it is one of the major entry points of prana into the body, particularly air prana. For this reason, it is always included in healing protocols for patients with infections.

The navel chakra is located directly on the belly button and, like the solar plexus chakra, controls many of the organs of the abdomen, including the large and small intestines. It also controls the birth process. It is often confused with the *tan tien*, ("field of elixir" or "field of chi") of Chinese and Taoist systems, or the *hara* of Japanese meditation and martial arts teachings. The tan tien (also spelled *dan tien*) is actually just below the navel chakra.

The meng mein chakra, or "gate of life," is located on the back, right between the kidneys. It governs the kidneys, adrenal glands, and partially the urinary system. The meng mein is an important pump and transformer, as it directs energy up the back of the spine from the basic chakra during meditation. Most significantly, for healing and meditation, it also controls the blood pressure. Thus, Pranic Healing treatments for hypertension always include the meng mein.

The sex chakra is situated right behind the pubic bone in both men and women. It energizes the legs, sex organs, and also the throat because, as noted previously, the sex chakra is the lower center of creativity and is thus connected to the higher center of creativity (throat chakra). The sex chakra also energizes the brain, as prana is regularly circulated through the body upward to the head.

The basic chakra, or "root," is located at the base of the spine. It governs the bones, muscles, soft tissue, and blood production. The basic chakra also affects your general sense of vitality and energy, the growth of children, and body temperature.

Together this aggregation of auras, chakras, and meridians—your energetic anatomy—has four main tasks:

1. It controls prana exchange or "pranic respiration"—that is, the regular intake and expelling of prana, as well as its circulation throughout the physical body.

2. With the chakras acting as transformers and regulators and the meridians functioning as wires, it modulates the level of prana throughout the physical body.

3. It acts as an energetic barrier for the physical body, protecting it against all the various types of energetic contamination to which it is subjected.

4. It acts as an "energetic pattern" for the physical body. People often believe the body contains the aura, but it is actually the other way around: the array of chakras and auras are actually the form for the physical body. This concept is better understood when presented in a more overtly spiritual context, and it's a topic worthy of a much longer discussion, but we'll summarize it very briefly here. The aura is the template for the physical body because of the esoteric or spiritual principle of correspondence, which states that there is an inner or energy world, and before something manifests in the physical world, it first manifests in that inner or energy world. Thus, the aura comes into being as the energetic manifestation of our divine nature, the Incarnated Soul mentioned in chapter 1. The nature of the Incarnated Soul is that it is pure, but not perfect. As a result, it continually strives to reconnect with the original source, God. This is the spiritual yearning that we all inherently possess. But in order for the soul to make progress toward reunification with God, it needs to incarnate first in a physical body to learn certain lessons. The most fundamental of these is to recognize our true nature—that we are spiritual beings having a human experience; that we are a soul first, and a physical body second. Thus, the Soul manifests in this material plane in the form that we know as a human being. And the aura provides the energetic pattern for that physical body.

TABLE 2.1 **THE ELEVEN MAJOR CHAKRAS**

CHAKRA	LOCATION	FUNCTIONS AND CORRESPONDING ORGANS	DISEASES
1. Crown	Crown of the head	Brain and pineal gland	Diseases related to pineal gland and brain (physical or psychological illnesses)
2. Forehead	Center of the forehead at the hairline	Nervous system and pineal gland	Loss of memory, paralysis, and epilepsy
3. Ajna	Between the eyebrows	Pituitary gland and endocrine glands; controls the other major chakras	Cancer, allergy, asthma, and diseases related to the endocrine glands
4. Throat	Center of the throat	Throat, thyroid and parathyroid glands	Throat-related illnesses such as goiter, sore throat, loss of voice, asthma, etc.
5. Heart a) Front heart	Center of the chest at the sternum	Heart, thymus gland, and circulatory system	Heart and circulatory ailments
b) Back heart	On the spine opposite the front heart chakra	Lungs, thymus gland, and to a lesser degree, the heart	Lung ailments
6. Solar plexus a) Front solar plexus	The hollow area just beneath sternum	Acts as an energy clearinghouse; also controls the heating and cooling of the body	Both front and back solar plexus: high cholesterol, diabetes, ulcer, hepatitis, rheumatoid arthritis, heart ailments, and other illnesses related to these organs
b) Back solar plexus	On the spine, opposite the front solar plexus chakra	Both front and back solar plexus: pancreas, liver, large and small intestine, appendix, and stomach	

CHAKRA	LOCATION	FUNCTIONS AND CORRESPONDING ORGANS	DISEASES
7. Spleen a) Front spleen b) Back spleen	Left part of the abdomen between front solar plexus chakra and navel; middle part of left bottom rib On the back, directly opposite the front spleen chakra	Both front and back spleen: major entry point for air prana; energize the other major chakras and the entire body	Both front and back spleen: low vitality, weak body, and blood ailments; autoimmune disorders
8. Navel	Navel	Small and large intestines	Constipation, difficulty in giving birth, appendicitis, low vitality, and other diseases related to intestines
9. Meng mein	Back of the navel	Kidneys, adrenal glands; energizes to a certain degree other internal organs; controls blood pressure	Kidney problems, low vitality, high blood pressure, and back problems
10. Sex	Behind the pubic bone	Sexual organs, bladder, and legs; lower or physical creative center	Sex-related and bladder problems
11. Basic	Base of the spine	Adrenal glands and sex organs; energizes the physical body—bones, muscles, blood, and internal organs; affects general vitality, body heat, and the growth of infants and children; center of self-survival or self-preservation	Cancer, leukemia, low vitality, allergy, asthma, sexual ailments, back problems, blood ailments, growth problems

Here's an analogy that may help you understand how your energetic anatomy relates to your physical body. If you squeeze a sponge dry, and then put it in a pot of water, it will absorb all the water it can hold and still be surrounded on all sides by water. The sponge is comparable to your body, and the water to your auras. The sponge both contains water and is surrounded by it, just as your physical body both contains prana and is surrounded by it. Thus, there is an interrelationship between the physical body and the energy body. That's why an illness can manifest first in the energy body before appearing as an affliction of the physical body. It's also why working on a health problem in the energy body, such as through Pranic Healing, can produce a healing of the physical body.

Seven vs. Eleven Chakras

Many people who come to Pranic Healing or Arhatic Yoga from other schools or who have read the "classic" Indian texts about prana, meditation, and spiritual development are surprised when they hear or read about references to eleven chakras. Most Aryan esoteric literature talks about seven chakras. The difference can be explained easily. If the school or training is focused primarily on spiritual development or enlightenment, then working with seven chakras will suffice, because the seven discussed are the traditional ones associated with the endocrine system: the basic or root, the spleen, the navel, the heart, the throat, the brow, and the crown. However, to be fully effective at physical healing, there are other significant energy centers in the body that need to be studied and understood. That's why Pranic Healing teaches students to work with eleven chakras. The other four are the sex chakra, the meng mein, the solar plexus, and the forehead. Also, most seven-chakra systems don't mention that the heart, solar plexus, and spleen have both a front and a back chakra. There are other healing systems that work with seven chakras—for instance, Reiki—but the four additional chakras help Pranic Healers properly access additional important organs and areas of the body that make its techniques particularly effective.

Other references to eleven chakras can be found in the Kabbalistic tradition, where the Tree of Life has eleven *sephiroth*, or attributes of God (actually ten, plus one hidden one), and the Upanishads, in which the Hindu deity Krishna speaks of the body as a "city with eleven gates."

THE FOUR KEYS TO EFFECTIVE ENERGY GENERATION

If you study or practice any of the more popular routines used to increase or balance personal energy or promote health, such as yoga, chi kung, or tai chi, movement-based programs such as Pilates or the Feldenkrais Method, and even some forms of breathwork, it's clear that these routines share a number of key characteristics that make them effective. Each employs these characteristics its own unique way, and so do the Nine Energizing Breaths. So before we move into the preparatory material and then to the actual step-by-step specifics of the Nine Energizing Breaths, let's briefly look at these key characteristics and how they come together in a particularly effective way in the routine in this book.

Breath Modification

The most basic observation that can be made about the energy that we call life force, regardless of the technique used to generate it or the cultural origin of the technique, is this: increasing energy begins with breathing, or with making the breathing more efficient. Whether it's called deep breathing, full breathing, natural breathing, yogic breathing, or—as you will learn it in the next chapter—pranic breathing, slower, deeper respiration is the fundamental building block for both physical relaxation and energy enhancement. The ancient cultures that developed such practices as yoga and tai chi chuan knew this as truth. The fact that the word for life force is synonymous with "air" or "breath" in so many of their languages is evidence of that. And now, the modern world—and even medical science—is rediscovering that connection. Deep breathing was cited as the second most popular alternative medicine treatment used by American adults, according to a 2007 survey by the National Institutes of Health's National Center for Complementary and Alternative Medicine.[2] And such leading medical facilities as the Palo Alto Center for Integrative Medicine in Stanford, California, and University Medical Center in Tucson, Arizona, have been offering seriously ill patients, including those with cancer and heart disease, access to breathing-based alternative treatments such as chi kung.[3]

One of the principal practices common to most forms of yoga is a series of elaborate breathing practices called *pranayama,* which is derived from the Sanskrit words *prana* ("life force" or "breath") and *ayama* ("length" or "expansion"). The idea is that the breath is modified by making the breath cycle of inspiration and expiration longer and slower (and in much higher levels of yoga, even stopping it completely); in so doing, practitioners relax their minds and bodies and increase their energy. As with yoga, there are many varieties of chi kung, but they all use some form of abdominal breathing and various breath modifications to increase the efficiency of our ability to draw in energy though respiration. Even many forms of the relatively modern healing practice called breathwork, a term that describes a range of therapeutic modalities that often have a person adjust his or her "normal" breathing pattern to access and release negative emotions held in the body's tissues, generate a surplus of prana through their breath modification techniques. So it's clear that increasing energy begins with breathing more effectively.

Physical Exercise, Movement, or Postures

The second element common to the most effective methods of producing an abundance of life force is some type of physical movement of the body—usually coordinated with breath modification. From basic aerobic exercise designed to increase endurance, to the static postures of yoga that increase flexibility, to the flowing, dancelike movements of tai chi chuan that enhance mind-body integration, it's clear that moving or positioning the body stimulates energy and breaks energetic blockages within the body. In most yoga styles, there is little dynamic movement; it typically involves fixed stances and slow bending and stretching. But many forms of yoga still contain subtle but very important movements for our internal physical and energetic anatomy. Certain postures squeeze, stimulate, twist, and exercise the endocrine glands and internal organs, which, in turn, clean the chakras associated with the glands and organs. In this way, energetic contamination is removed from the aura, and fresh prana is drawn in.

Chi kung was devised by and for Taoist monks to generate energy for enlightenment and higher-level spiritual development, and it originally consisted of mostly breathing exercises in still or seated meditative postures. However, when the Buddhist Ta Mo traveled to China from India and introduced yoga-type physical exercises to the breathing routine, the system in the Taoist temples became fully developed—and capable of creating even more energy. As a result, the generally weak and sickly frames of the monks became greatly strengthened.

While the movements of the most popular styles of tai chi chuan are slow and graceful, they are coordinated with breathing for two purposes: first, to relax what ancient Chinese scholars called our "monkey mind," the nature of the mind to flit from thought to thought the way a jittery monkey jumps from limb to limb in a tree; and second, to maximize the production of chi to defeat an opponent in combat. (Even though most people today practice tai chi chuan for health and energy reasons, it's important to remember it was developed as a fighting art.)

Many forms of breathwork exercise the muscles of the torso, and especially the diaphragm, to help release negative emotional tension often held there. It is this physical movement of the breathing—moving the diaphragm up and down through its full range of motion—together with the breathing itself, that helps relax the mind and body, as well as free up the energy frequently blocked there.

In summary, moving the body in some purposeful way is helpful for producing large quantities of prana.

Application of Mind

Along with breathing and movement, some type of mind focus—in the form of intent, concentration, will, or visualization—is often used to relax the body and enhance the production of life force or to guide this energy to wherever you want the energy to go. Chinese systems probably include more overt instruction for applying the mind (intent and visualization) to exercises and breathing than other systems. In tai chi chuan and chi kung training, there is a popular saying, "The chi follows the yi." The chi, of course, is your energy, your prana. *Yi* roughly translates as "mind" or "intent." Thus, students are taught that their energy will go where they intend it to go, if they lightly direct it. But will and visualization certainly have their place in yoga as well, and in much the same way as expressed in the Chinese adage above. Some forms of breathwork urge you to focus on a particular area in order to clear out negative emotional energy; others simply suggest you allow the clearing of negative emotions to happen without willful direction. And of course, many of these systems contain techniques for using the mind or visualization to consciously relax the body and thus allow and direct the energy to flow better through the body.

Meditation

Meditation is an integral part of many forms of yoga and chi kung, and tai chi chuan is often called a "moving meditation." We don't often think of breathwork as a type of formal meditation, but if meditation is defined as a state in which the body and mind reach a sufficient state of relaxation so that there is minimal differentiation between them, then certainly many types of breathwork produce a meditative state. Even physical exercise can produce that meditative state. Runners speak of a "runner's high," and athletes talk about being "in the zone," a state of peak performance where they feel fully integrated with their bodies, and time appears to slows down so that they can perform effortlessly. Athletes also often say they perform unconsciously—and at their best—in such a state.

Certain meditations can be highly conducive to increasing life force in three ways: first, those that relax the body and mind (such as a breath awareness or mindfulness meditation), calm our monkey mind, and thus facilitate the smooth circulation of prana throughout the energy body because there is less tension and resistance in the aura; second, many meditations promote deep or pranic breathing, which automatically generates life force; and third, some meditations actually enable the practitioner to draw down through the crown chakra very high-quality prana, which can then be used to clean and energize the aura.

THE KEY CHARACTERISTICS OF SUCCESSFUL ENHANCEMENT OF LIFE FORCE AND THE NINE ENERGIZING BREATHS

Here is how these four key characteristics are integrated into the Nine Energizing Breaths: before you learn the Nine Energizing Breaths, you will first learn pranic breathing, which is deep abdominal breathing coupled with a number of highly advanced but simple-to-perform *breath modifications* that will turbocharge your energy-building capacity. Both pranic breathing and the Nine Energizing Breaths utilize the principles of *rhythm* and *retention,* which are simply breathing in and out to a certain count while holding or "retaining" the breath at select points in each breath cycle. These special rhythms and breath pauses are the key to building up large quantities of prana. Additionally, each of the Nine Energizing Breaths has a specific breathing pattern that cleans and energizes either a particular portion of your aura or your entire aura.

There are two important ways that you will blend *physical movement* into the Nine Energizing Breaths program. First, you will learn the Cleansing Physical Exercises, a specially designed set of simple twists and stretches that helps break up the energetic blockages in your aura that can lead to musculoskeletal tension, stress, and even physical ailments in your body. It's recommended that you perform them prior to meditation and the Nine Energizing Breaths. Before meditation, the Cleansing Physical Exercises help loosen and stretch the physical body, which also loosens and stretches the chakras. This helps discharge stagnant or dirty prana from the aura and also prepares the aura to accept the additional, fresh prana accumulated during meditation. After meditation, the Cleansing Physical Exercises can be used to disperse from the physical and energetic bodies any pranic congestion built up by your meditative practice. (Most meditations, even mild ones such as simple mindfulness practice, generate prana in the aura. If the aura isn't sufficiently prepared to assimilate the prana—usually because the aura isn't clean enough—the meditator can experience a variety of physical symptoms. These include anxiety, physical discomfort, muscular tension, and most often, drowsiness. But physical exercise following meditation helps discharge this prana and avoid these physical symptoms.) Second, when you perform the Nine Energizing Breaths, you will use precise physical movements while applying a specific breathing pattern. Each action or motion of the routine moves or pushes the prana through a certain series of meridians and chakras in the body.

The *application of mind* is very important in the Nine Energizing Breaths, as you will have to establish your "intent" at the outset of each exercise. Perhaps even more important, you will learn that intent isn't jaw-clenched concentration or the teeth-gritting willpower you use to force out one more repetition when you lift weights. That sort of strong will has its place in life, but it's actually counterproductive to the plentiful production of prana because it creates tension in the physical and energy body, which inhibits the smooth flow of prana. Rather, you will learn that intent is merely "light awareness," or gently focused attention, on the breathing routine and bodily movements you're performing to develop maximum energy. Here's how to distinguish between *will* and *intent*: place your right thumb into the middle of your left palm. Really push it in for a few seconds so that when you take it away, you can still feel the pressure and even see the imprint on your skin. Afterward, regardless of whether you bring your attention to your left palm or not, you're still aware of that pressure sensation. That type of thumb pressure is focusing your will. Now take your right index finger and gently tap the middle of your left palm three times. If you turn your attention back to what you were doing before you started this exercise—reading a book, watching television, typing at your computer—you won't feel your left palm. But if you close your eyes and breathe quietly, letting your thoughts go, you can feel a slight sensation remaining in your left palm. That light tapping is intent.

Finally, while *meditation* isn't essential to the Nine Energizing Breaths, it is a wonderful complement. Chapter 7 includes three simple but powerful meditations, including the very special Meditation on Twin Hearts, which will help you open your heart and crown chakras through the practice of loving-kindness and mindfulness. At the same time, it also draws down large quantities of prana through your crown chakra. But here's why the Nine Energizing Breaths help you maximize your meditation practice: after you finish one of the three meditations in this book, or any meditation, the prana you generate will filter through and move around your aura for a little while, and then eventually dissipate as you return to your normal worldly activities. However, when you perform the Nine Energizing Breaths immediately after meditation, its special breathing patterns and body locks help to "physicalize," or infuse into the body's tissues, the high-quality energy you generate during meditation. As a result, the prana actually stays in the physical body much longer rather than dispersing, and after a period of time practicing the Nine Energizing Breaths following meditation, your physical body becomes saturated with prana. Performed diligently, this routine can begin to reverse the aging process, leading to a more youthful appearance.

* * *

As mentioned earlier, there are many styles of yoga, martial arts (such as tai chi chuan or chi kung), and other practices that can be used quite effectively to increase your energy, but the Nine Energizing Breaths are generally easier to learn and perform. They also take less time, while still generating a tremendous amount of energy. We certainly don't want to disparage any other systems, because the Nine Energizing Breaths are, in many ways, a compilation of the best of yoga, chi kung, and other energy-generating practices. They're just easier to practice—and the benefits can be seen immediately.

For instance, the movements of tai chi chuan may be simple to perform physically, but they actually demand a high degree of focus and practice, and it takes time to master the forms. Many yoga postures require a degree of flexibility or athleticism the average person may find difficult to attain. There are some chi kung styles that can increase your energy quite dramatically, but they're often complex and lengthy, or they can be dangerous to practice without the personal guidance of a qualified teacher. (This is also true of many types of yoga, particularly kundalini yoga.) Even certain types of breathwork can release pent-up emotional energy suddenly and dramatically, which can be startling—and even frightening—to the practitioner, so direct, supported guidance is often needed with advanced forms of breathwork.

The difference with the Nine Energizing Breaths is that you are *not* required to do any of the following:

- Be particularly athletic, strong, or flexible
- Study personally with a master or teacher
- Perform complex postures
- Learn complicated breathing routines

They simply enable you to consciously, actively, dynamically—and safely—enhance your personal supply of energy, of prana, with minimal training and in just a few minutes a day. And when you do this, you have at your disposal a powerful routine to boost your energy and revitalize your body.

Chapter 3   The Importance of Pranic Breathing

Margie Ramsey is a nurse in a busy Los Angeles hospital who uses the Nine Energizing Breaths to keep her going throughout a hectic day. She estimates that her energy "almost doubles" after performing the routine only one time, and she reports that "even my sense of physical balance improves" as she practices them. Margie also finds them "easy and fun to do" and says, "It's an exercise that anyone can do at any age." Whenever she performs the Nine Energizing Breaths, she says, "I can feel the results right away."

We all understand how important breath is to life. Most people have heard some variation of the following: a person can live ten days or more without food, and about three days without water, but only four to five minutes without breathing, before nerve cells begin to die and there is a loss of brain and organ function that may be irreversible. This is all true. Yet notice how we usually understand the importance of breathing only as a biological process—that is, oxygenating the blood and expelling carbon dioxide. There is actually another aspect to breathing besides the physiological, and that's the energetic; for breathing is our primary means of drawing in not only oxygen but also prana or life force. As you read in the previous chapter, our body extracts this vital life force automatically as we breathe. But in order to boost your energy, to increase the quantity of your life force and move your energy exchange level from unconscious and passive to conscious and active, you need to learn to breathe "properly."

"PROPER" BREATHING

Most people would be surprised if you told them they weren't breathing properly. After all, breathing is instinctive. Why would you need someone to teach you how to breathe "properly"? Your body knows how to breathe quite well. Well, yes, breathing is performed unconsciously, the same way drawing in a baseline amount of prana is carried out unconsciously. But the truth is, most people do breathe inefficiently and improperly—at least in regard to the type of breathing needed to draw in great quantities of prana to energize themselves. In fact, learning to breathe properly is the first and easiest step you can take toward increasing your overall energy level. Simple to learn and master, proper breathing will quickly deliver numerous benefits. Among the physiological benefits, to name just a few: an increase in lung capacity, more efficient oxygen exchange, improved endurance, better cardiovascular functioning, diminished musculoskeletal tension, physical relaxation, mental relaxation, and anxiety reduction. Among the energetic benefits: a cleaner energy body, straightened health rays in the aura, an increased capacity to take in and utilize large quantities of high-quality prana, and release of negative emotions held in the body.

Rather than breathing properly—that is, drawing in a full, slow, silent breath down to the bottom of their lungs—most people breathe "high" and "shallow." This means they breathe not by moving their abdomen out and in but by moving their chest and ribs out and in and their collarbones up and down. Additionally, most people breathe too quickly. The average breathing rate is twelve to sixteen cycles (inhalations and exhalations) per minute—which is actually on the verge of hyperventilation. When your breathing is high, shallow, and rapid, you reduce the amount of oxygen you draw into your lungs—and the amount of prana you take in. Additionally, this "self-manufactured" oxygen shortage will trigger, in many people, the body's fight-or-flight reflex, which causes a whole cascade of physiological, biochemical, and energetic changes: your body releases a flood of hormones such as adrenaline and cortisol that prepare you to physically defend yourself or run away. This, in turn, increases your muscle tension and anxiety, which also decreases your energy. (Technically, the fight-or-flight impulse increases your energy, as the body prepares to defend itself against a perceived assault or danger. However, this isn't relaxing energy; it's a high-tension spike of nervous energy that is inevitably followed by an energy crash, similar to the crash following a couple cups of coffee. That's why you feel so exhausted after going through an emotionally taxing ordeal. Your body has had a hormonally driven surge of energy that can't be sustained.)

Thus the cycle of poor breathing, tension, and low energy is established. We breathe improperly, which creates tension, which leads to the body releasing stress hormones. And of course when we are tense, we either hold our breath or breathe more shallowly or irregularly, which leads to greater tension, more stress hormones in the bloodstream, and in time, an establishment of the fight-or-flight reflex as our normal condition. With poor breathing, we create our own feedback loop to keep us in a state of constant stress and low energy, and thus poor breathing reduces both our physiological and our energetic potential.

Now, we don't start out breathing improperly; in fact, it's learned behavior. Every baby breathes instinctively from the abdomen, which you can see if you watch small children and babies when they're asleep. As we get older, however, tension and the effects of stress on the body inhibit our natural breathing process. As discussed in the introduction, we are prone to holding negative emotions such as fear, stress, and anger, plus limiting beliefs and traumatic memories, as tension in the musculature of our bodies. And the muscles throughout the torso are one of the main places we store that tension. This includes the diaphragm, the tough, flat, oval muscle that lies under the lungs and that is drawn down when the lungs inflate fully; the intercostal muscles, which are the small, thin muscles between and supporting the ribcage; and the smooth muscle of the lung tissue itself. Tightness in any of these areas, as you can imagine, makes it difficult to draw a full breath.

We also have tension throughout the chest and torso because we don't stretch and exercise the area properly. Today's emphasis on fitness and muscle tone is definitely positive. But many people place more importance on size and musculature than on flexibility. Bench presses, overhead presses, chin-ups, and other upper-body exercises create bigger and stronger muscles in the chest, arms, and shoulders, but they decrease flexibility in those areas if these exercises are not supplemented with regular stretching. And most people don't stretch sufficiently and often enough. Surprisingly, the current desire for "washboard abs" also creates torso tension. When you exercise the abdominals and condition yourself to holding your stomach in to keep it flat, you are actually training yourself to be a chest rather than abdominal breather because you keep the lower abdomen pulled in and tight.

"Proper" Breathing Now Viewed as a Legitimate Health and Energy Aid

Interestingly, the act of breathing has begun to be recognized by the traditional medical establishment as a tremendous help to health and overall energy. Consider these examples: The FDA has approved breath training as a treatment for high blood pressure.[1] A study at Wayne State University School of Medicine in Detroit revealed that menopausal women who practiced what the researchers called yogic "belly breathing" reduced the frequency of their hot flashes by 50 percent.[2] Noted alternative medicine pioneer Andrew Weil, MD, teaches proper breathing to all his patients and has said that breathing is "the simplest and most powerful technique for protecting your health."[3] And James Gordon, MD, another well-known mind-body medicine advocate, has been quoted as saying that "slow, deep breathing is probably the single best anti-stress medicine we have. . . . [It] gives people a sense of control over their body and their emotions that is extremely therapeutic."[4]

PRANIC BREATHING

So that you're clear on the difference between high, shallow, and rapid breathing, on one hand, and "proper" or, as we call it here, pranic breathing,[5] on the other, let's do a quick comparison. Lie down on the floor or any firm surface (just not a soft bed). Loosen your belt, if you're wearing one. Place your right hand on your chest and your left hand on your abdomen, with your palm over your navel. Breathe normally for about sixty seconds, and be aware of the movement of your hands, chest, and stomach. For most people, their chests, rather than their abdomens, will move. This is high and shallow breathing.

Now, let's learn pranic breathing.

Exercise 3.1 **Pranic Breathing**

1. You may close your eyes or keep them open throughout this exercise, whichever is more comfortable for you. Sit on the edge of a chair, sofa, or bed, but keep your back straight and away from the back of the chair or sofa. Place both thumbs on your navel and spread your hands across your lower belly.

2. Put your tongue on the roof of your mouth just behind the hard palate (the hard ridge behind your top row of teeth), and keep it there as you breathe. This connects the two major meridians, or energy channels, in your body and facilitates the flow of prana. One meridian runs down the front of the body from the palate to the perineum. This is called the "conception" or "main" meridian. The other runs from the perineum up along the spine, over the back of the head, down the forehead, and terminates at the top of the palate. This is called the "governor" meridian.

3. Exhale through your mouth until your lungs are comfortably empty, but don't strain. Your stomach should move in, but try to keep your spine straight.

4. Begin breathing in slowly and silently through your nose. Feel your lungs filling up in three segments—first the top one-third, then the middle one-third, and finally, the bottom one-third. Your chest should not move as you breathe in, only your abdomen. As your lungs reach capacity, pause for a moment; then exhale smoothly and gently through your nose. This completes one cycle of pranic breathing. Try it again up to ten times. Rest for a few minutes; then do ten more breaths. If you feel dizzy or uncomfortable at all, stop immediately and just breathe regularly for a few minutes before resuming.

Most people master the coordination of pranic breathing in less than two weeks.

SUPPLEMENTAL EXERCISES TO FACILITATE PRANIC BREATHING

If you're having difficulty getting the mechanics of pranic breathing down, there are a couple of exercises that may help. Each was designed by noted therapist and breathwork expert Gay Hendricks, PhD. The first will address any tension in your torso by helping you loosen up your diaphragm. The second will help you keep your focus lower in the abdomen rather than higher up in your chest as you breathe.

Exercise 3.2 **Loosening Your Torso and Diaphragm**
1. Lie down on your back on a firm surface, with your knees up and feet flat on the ground.

2. Take a full, deep abdominal breath (though don't strain); then hold it gently.

3. While holding the breath in, suck in your abdomen, moving your navel back toward your spine. Your diaphragm will move up into your chest, and your ribcage will move up slightly as you do this.

4. Hold this position for a second, and while still holding your breath, relax and push your abdomen back out, allowing it to bulge.

5. Keep this position for a second, and while still holding your breath, repeat the suck in/bulge out sequence again. See if you can do a set of up to ten repetitions while holding your breath.

6. Eventually you will find it easy to do up to thirty repetitions of this movement during one held breath. What this exercise does is force the diaphragm to move up and down, increasing its mobility. It also allows some gentle stretching and relaxation of the muscles at the front and sides of the abdomen.

Exercise 3.3 Keeping Your Focus on Your Abdomen Rather Than Your Chest

1. Lie down on your back on a firm surface. Your legs can be bent at the knee or extended straight out.

2. Place a book on your navel. It should be heavy enough that you can feel its weight without being too uncomfortable. A heavy hardcover book without the dust jacket works best.

3. Now, begin pranic breathing as you learned in the previous exercises, breathing slowly, evenly, and deeply. The book should rise and fall with each breath. If the book does not move, try a heavier book until you can feel your abdominal area.

4. Take your time. When you can tell you're getting your breath deep into your abdomen, do the exercise without the book. If, at any time, you lose the feeling, simply put the book back.

Observations on Chest Breathers and Diaphragmatic Tension in Patients

Almost without exception, the sickest patients I see in my practice all breathe high up in the chest. I have been studying breathing patterns in my patients for years, and I can honestly say that no more than three to five adult patients out of the roughly four thousand I see annually are breathing correctly. Is there a connection between improper breathing and illness, and between proper breathing and health? Psychologist Gay Hendricks, PhD, cites a study in his book *Conscious Breathing* (see Further Reading) of twenty-five first-time heart attack victims in the Netherlands. The patients were divided into two groups. The first group was taught abdominal breathing, while the second received no special training. At a two-year follow-up, seven of the twelve patients who were not taught diaphragmatic breathing had been readmitted for second heart attacks. None of the thirteen patients in the other group had further heart attacks during the study period.

I must say, my own clinical practice validates Hendricks's study, because the groups I've observed with the most shallow breathing have been, ironically, heart patients and asthmatics. Yet there are probably no groups that would benefit more from learning abdominal or pranic breathing.

Additionally, whenever I work with someone who is suffering from either anxiety or depression—and that is one of the most frequent problems I see, even in patients with more specific "physical" symptoms—I know their breathing is going to be very shallow and very high up in the chest. And I immediately introduce them to pranic breathing, the same exercises we're presenting here.

Between negative emotions and shallow breathing, it's difficult to say which is the cause and which is the effect. That's because holding stress in your chest or abdomen creates shallow breathing, and shallow breathing, in turn, can worsen anxiety and depression. But I have seen that deep abdominal breathing without a doubt can significantly reduce feelings of anxiety and depression. Here's an example: a forty-year-old nurse in one of our medical clinics was going through some marital problems, and as a result she was having frequent bouts of depression as well as anxiety attacks. As with most people undergoing stressful life events, her breathing was shallow and high. I taught her pranic breathing, and she started performing it regularly. After two weeks of practice, her diaphragm finally loosened up, and as it did, she reported that the frequency and the severity of her attacks were each reduced by about 90 percent. After the initial two weeks, she did the breathing as needed whenever she felt anxiety or depression coming on, and the exercises stopped the feelings before they could become physical symptoms. She also taught the breathing techniques to her daughter, who was undergoing the typical stresses of an adolescent girl, and she reported that her daughter's general anxiety was significantly reduced as well.

ERIC B. ROBINS, MD

The mechanics of pranic breathing are simple to learn and even master with minimal daily practice. However, there are some nuances that you can add to your practice to make it easier and more effective. For instance, breathe in and out through the nose rather than the mouth. From a purely physiological perspective, this is more effective for you because nose hairs filter out small particles of dust and dirt. The baffles and channels of the nose also warm up the air, which makes it easier to assimilate the prana. But from an energetic perspective, when you breathe in and out through the nose, you not only cleanse the aura and physical body, you also keep the fresh prana you accumulate during breathing in the aura. When you breathe in through the nose and out through the mouth—and there are exercises for which this is appropriate—it has a stronger expelling effect, and you're cleansing more than energizing the aura and physical body. Beginning students often ask about the level of effort they should put into their practice. Your breathing should be smooth and easy, almost effortless. As you start out, the muscles of your torso may prevent you from breathing deeply from your diaphragm, but simply stick with your practice, and they will loosen up. But don't consciously try to slow down your breathing; let it happen. There is an ancient saying from chi kung practice regarding breathing that is instructive about the appropriate effort. Chinese masters said breathing should be "slow, slim, silent, and slender." Breathing that is rushed or forced can be none of these. And finally, don't practice on a full stomach. Within an hour or two after eating, your body is focused on digestion, and you may be a big groggy. It's better to practice your breathing thirty minutes before or two hours after a meal.

BOOSTING THE POWER OF YOUR BREATHING: RHYTHM AND RETENTION[6]

Breathing rhythm is just what it sounds like: the pace of your in-breath and out-breath. You can find breathing rhythms in activities such as tai chi chuan, meditation, self-hypnosis, martial arts, and breathwork, to name just a few. Each of these routines has its own unique breathing rhythms, but they all use them in similar ways. For instance, many forms of self-hypnosis advise the subject to sit quietly and relax the body one part at a time, while breathing slowly in and out at a certain pace. There are many meditations that begin with the subject directed to "watch" or "be aware" of the breath and its natural rhythm. And tai chi chuan practitioners are instructed to breathe normally but slowly, to establish a soft, easy rhythm. In these instances, and in many others, we see that one of the most universal attributes of a breathing rhythm is its power to induce relaxation, to calm and clear the mind. However, it isn't widely known that some unique breathing rhythms actually can do more than relax you; they can boost the power of your breathing, enabling you to draw in greater supplies of prana. You'll learn several of those breathing patterns here.

Breathing retention is pausing and holding your breath briefly at the end of each inhalation and exhalation. Holding your breath after exhalation is called *empty retention*, and holding it after inhalation is called *full retention*. In yoga, breath retention is called *kumbhaka*, which means "vessel," "pitcher," or "pot." When you hold your breath momentarily, you are filling up your vessel, your energy body, with prana. Empty retention is called *bahya kumbhaka*, and full retention is called *antara kumbhaka*. In yogic terms, the inhalation is called *puraka*, or "act of filling," and the exhalation is called *rechaka*, or "act of emptying." In Pranic Healing, we simply say that breath retention creates an "energetic bellows effect." You pump a set of bellows rhythmically to strengthen the flame in a fireplace. In the same way, holding your breath for a moment boosts your prana generation.

The rhythm and retention patterns you will learn here act as "pranic turbochargers," intensifying the prana's healthful effects and driving the prana vigorously throughout your energy body. We often show Pranic Healing students a simple way to illustrate how rhythm and retention increase the power of pranic breathing exponentially. One person stands in the front of the room breathing normally, while others stand around the first student and scan, or actually feel the size, strength, and contours of the person's aura. Before pranic breathing, most people who are healthy have an aura that extends out about six inches all around their physical bodies. But as the person begins pranic breathing, the scanners feel the aura grow stronger and even more solid. Many report that it feels like holding the north end of one magnet against the north end of another magnet; their hands feel resistance. It's not unusual for scanners to feel the aura push out to twenty or thirty feet, or even more, if the person continues to perform pranic breathing.

PRANIC BREATHING: THE KEY TO BOTH RELAXATION AND ENERGY

Here's why pranic breathing both invigorates and calms you. When you are under stress, your breathing becomes shallow and irregular, largely because the muscles of the torso—principally, the diaphragm—become tense and unable to move through their entire range. You breathe higher up in the chest and don't draw breaths deep into the lungs. We are thus told to "breathe deeply" during times of stress in order to loosen the diaphragm and get it working through its full range. That's the physiological explanation as to why deep breathing helps relax you. But there's an energetic reason as well. Your energy is at its optimal level and your mind is calmest when your chakras spin in sync—that is, at a similar, though not necessarily exact, speed, spinning smoothly, alternating between clockwise and counterclockwise. When they spin clockwise, they draw in fresh energy; when they spin counterclockwise, they expel dirty energy. In a healthy person, there is a coordination or synchronization among the chakras as they perform these energizing and expelling functions; they work in a state of dynamic equilibrium, a delicate balance that's constantly adjusting. However, this delicate balance can be disrupted for a variety of reasons. For instance, when you are stressed, you often hold the tension, as noted earlier, in the torso, which causes the throat, front heart, front solar plexus, and navel chakras to slow down and/or to spin erratically. If you are frequently angry, anxious, or fearful, these negative emotions will knock your chakras out of sync. And if you eat an energetically unclean diet (see chapter 4), your navel and solar plexus chakras are likely to be frequently congested and spin unevenly. When the chakras spin erratically or work out of sync, the smooth flow of prana throughout your energetic anatomy is disrupted, and you can have areas of energetic congestion and depletion. This makes the physical body more prone to physical and emotional ailments.

But slow, rhythmic pranic breathing helps remedy all these situations. It relaxes the muscles of the torso, restores flexibility to the diaphragm, and enables the chakras to become synchronized. The result is a calming effect, as well as a buildup of energy. Pranic breathing thus helps you both to relax and to energize, to stay tranquil and to stay alert—which is a pretty good way to go through your daily activities!

In yogic thinking, life is measured not according to the number of years lived but according to the number of breaths taken in that lifetime. This gives us a better understanding of why yoga places so much emphasis on slowing down and on controlling or holding the breath. In yoga, the formal practice of breath control is called pranayama, which, as noted earlier, is derived from the words *prana* ("life force" or "breath") and *ayama* ("length" or "expansion"). Of course, this is also an extension of yogic philosophy's understanding of the connection between breathing, energy, health, and well-being. In increasing the length of the breath and the number of breaths taken, as well as holding the breath in certain ways, the yoga practitioner calms the mind, generates more prana, and increases his or her lifespan.

Exercise 3.4 Optimum Pranic Breathing Rhythm and Retention: 7-1-7-1

There are many different systems that teach breathing rhythm as a method of increasing energy or promoting relaxation. The 7-1-7-1 taught in Pranic Healing and Arhatic Yoga was determined through clairvoyant observation to be the optimum for those starting out their breathing practice. It's easy to remember and thus practice. But it also produces a significant amount of energy.

(Note: If you have hypertension, don't hold your breath longer than one second. Pranic breathing stimulates all the chakras, and especially the navel and the meng mein. The meng mein controls the blood pressure, and if you hold your breath too long, it could unsafely increase your blood pressure.)

1. Put your tongue on your palate and keep it there as you breathe.

2. Inhale for 7 counts, in the pranic breathing manner you learned in exercise 3.1.

3. Hold for 1 count.

4. Exhale for 7 counts.

5. Hold for 1 count.

This five-step process is one cycle of pranic breathing. At the outset of your practice, try to do two or three sets of ten cycles daily. Take a minute or two between sets initially; then shorten the length of your rest time as you progress. With practice, you won't need to consciously count off the rhythm in your mind. You can begin by using one second per count; however, the length of the counts is not as important as maintaining the ratio and the steady pace. As you progress, you may find that your heartbeat is an effective pacing mechanism, too. If you're prone to anxiety, this will also help you reduce your heart rate.

Exercise 3.5 A More Powerful Rhythm and Retention Routine: 6-3-6-3

After you practice the 7-1-7-1 routine for a while, and you get used to the energy it produces, try a rhythm of 6-3-6-3. It's stronger and produces more prana. As a result, it's the rhythm and retention used by most pranic healers and more advanced students in Grandmaster Choa's classes. However, after you practice both, feel free to use the one that's easier and more effective for you.

1. Place your tongue on your palate and keep it there as you breathe.

2. Inhale for 6 counts, in the pranic breathing manner you learned in exercise 3.1.

3. Hold for 3 counts.

4. Exhale for 6 counts.

5. Hold for 3 counts.

Again, try to perform two or three sets of ten cycles daily. As you practice, your energy-generation ability will compound, and your energy will increase exponentially.

When some more experienced students coming into Grandmaster Choa's classes learn about pranic breathing, they often inquire whether they should perform them using "regular" or "reverse" abdominal breathing. Regular abdominal breathing is allowing the abdomen to expand outward as you breathe in and compress as you breathe out. Reverse abdominal breathing is just what the name states: you pull the abdomen in as you breathe in and push it out as you breathe out. It's a much more aggressive form of breathing often learned in Chinese martial arts systems, such as tai chi chuan combat styles, and we don't recommend it.

Reverse abdominal breathing compresses the prana or chi that you generate into a smaller physical space in your body. It also stimulates the adrenal glands and the key lower chakras that are responsible for physical strength: the navel, meng mein, and basic chakras. The purpose is to create more energy in these lower chakras so that it can then be transmitted up through the body to the arms and hands in order to strike an opponent with greater force.

Overstimulating the lower chakras—particularly the meng mein, as you do in reverse abdominal breathing—can lead to an excess of "hot" energy that can literally wear out the body and lead to premature death due to heart attack or stroke. (In Taoist philosophy, martial arts, and traditional Chinese medicine, hot energy is *yang*; it is hard or strong energy for exertion, and it comes primarily from the ground. Hot energy is associated with the lower chakras. "Cool" or "cold" energy is *yin*; it is a complement and balance to hard energy, and it comes primarily from above. Cool or cold energy is associated with the upper chakras.) In Chinese, meng mein is "the gate of life" because it is a pumping station that pushes energy from the lower chakras up to the head. But it also regulates circulation and blood pressure. Thus, when you consistently overenergize the lower chakras, you also put undue stress upon your circulation system. In older times in Chinese tai chi chuan circles, those who practiced yang-style tai chi chuan, the gentle, flowing exercise routine that most of us today are familiar with, often lived into their eighties. Yang style emphasizes regular abdominal breathing. Those who practiced the more aggressive *chen*-style tai chi chuan, a system designed for combat, often bragged of having so much energy that they slept only several hours per night and had extremely powerful fighting ability, but they frequently lived only into their forties or fifties. Chen style employs reverse abdominal breathing. The goal in the Nine Energizing Breaths program is to gently stimulate your production of prana while synchronizing your chakras and calming your mind and body so that you have all the energy you need to live your life fully. The goal isn't to increase your energy to the degree that you don't need sleep or rest. That is unwise and unsafe.

PRACTICE

As you begin to develop your regular practice routine, keep in mind your goals and the time you have available. It's more effective to your long-term development—and health—to get in a couple of good practice sessions a week than it is to rush through a sloppy session daily. The goal of more energy is important, but it's also a journey of personal development, and you should enjoy that experience. You won't enjoy it if you turn it into a daily chore, or it becomes one more item on your already busy to-do list. With that as a guideline, here is a sample practice schedule. During your first week of practice, perform one to three sets of ten cycles of pranic breathing daily, using your own rhythm. During the second week, perform one to three sets of ten cycles of pranic breathing daily, using the 7-1-7-1 rhythm. During week three, perform one to three sets of ten cycles of pranic breathing daily, using the 6-3-6-3 rhythm. After three weeks, you should have a pretty good mastery of both the 7-1-7-1 and the 6-3-6-3 routines, so just vary your practice and rhythm according to your schedule and interest.

Chapter 4   Energetic Hygiene

Jasmine Marie Dickens learned the Nine Energizing Breaths during a Basic Pranic Healing class in Los Angeles. Before beginning the routine, she described herself as feeling physically tired. "I was a bit hungry, so my energy felt a bit lower than usual," she said. Since she was also "detoxing from a transition in my life," Jasmine was feeling emotionally drained as well. After performing just one set of the Nine Energizing Breaths, she said, "I was immediately energized," reporting a 25 percent increase in her energy level. She also calls the exercises a "wonderful facilitator for meditation."

For proper auto maintenance, the coolant in your car's radiator should be changed at regular intervals. Occasionally, you can just add a little water or antifreeze, simply topping it off and replacing the fluid that has evaporated due to day-to-day driving. But to make sure your engine runs at peak performance, you should get regularly what is called a "power flush," in which the dirty coolant is forcibly pushed through the radiator, engine, and hoses to get all the dirt, rust, and corrosion out of your cooling system. Then, the fresh coolant that you add can work much more efficiently.

If you think of your aura as a car radiator, you'll understand the importance of Energetic Hygiene, which is the practice of keeping your personal energy tank clean and full.[1] Your aura, like your car radiator, can generally handle the day-to-day "energetic contamination" that we encounter by virtue of living in a world with the many sources of environmental and emotional toxicity that you read about in chapter 2. However, when we are subjected to higher or repeated levels of contamination—through such things as living in a highly polluted area or experiencing stressful life events—the chakras and meridians can become depleted or congested, and the aura unbalanced. Thus, in order to keep the *quality* of your prana high, the aura also needs to be flushed regularly. This is best accomplished by consistently practicing good Energetic Hygiene.

Put another way, just as we bathe or shower daily for physical hygiene, we need to clean our aura daily—or at least regularly—in order to have good Energetic Hygiene. When you practice good Energetic Hygiene, you are also following another one of the basic rules of energy work and healing, which is to clean or purify before energizing. In a Pranic Healing treatment, the congested or depleted chakras or ailing areas of the body are first "swept," or cleaned of any dirty energy. Then they are energized with fresh prana. You're applying the same principle to increasing your own personal energy supply when you practice Energetic Hygiene.

Additionally, since an ailment will manifest first as an energetic disturbance in the aura before appearing as a physical illness in the body, keeping the aura as clean as possible through proper and regular Energetic Hygiene helps keep you healthier—mentally, emotionally, and physically. Problems don't even get a chance to take root in your aura, let alone in your body.

HOW TO KEEP YOUR ENERGY CLEAN IN A CONTAMINATED WORLD

In a world where people often have stressful jobs that aggravate them, live in cities where there may be a high level of residual contamination, and have to interact with people who may not always be positive and have at least some unresolved negative emotions, how *do* you keep your personal energy supply clean and full? In short, how do you maintain good Energetic Hygiene in a world full of contamination?

One proven way would be to live like the monks and gurus of old. Followed scrupulously, that lifestyle would enable you to lead a life fairly free of modern stressors, a life of energetic cleanliness and personal energy potency. But you'd probably have to move to a cave in the mountains, or at least away from cities. You'd also have to focus most of your waking hours on proper food preparation, breathing, meditating, and energy-generating exercises. Few people today would be willing to do that. (And to be perfectly candid, neither would we!)

The true key to good Energetic Hygiene in an energetically imperfect world is to realize simply that we do live in a contaminated world, and then to opt for the most healthful, energetically clean choices when you are able to, without getting too extreme or rigid in your approach. That's the approach Grandmaster Choa advocated, that's the approach we take personally, and that's what we recommend in this book. Practice Energetic Hygiene regularly—but moderately. Incorporate as much of this routine into your life as you can—and as you are personally comfortable doing. Don't lose sleep over it. We are definitely not fanatics.

So here are three of the simplest and most powerful Energetic Hygiene techniques taught to Arhatic Yoga and Pranic Healing students: a few dietary recommendations, cutting energetic cords, and utilizing the cleansing power of salt. Although Energetic Hygiene is a large topic worthy of far more space than we can devote to it here, and there are many other more complex Energetic Hygiene techniques, these three basic practices, if done regularly, will enable you to achieve a very high degree of energetic cleanliness.

DIETARY RECOMMENDATIONS

In order to maintain good Energetic Hygiene with your diet, the rule is simple: eat closer to the primary sources of energy. This means eating more fruits, vegetables, and whole grains, all of which get their prana directly from those primary sources: the air, sun, water, and earth (soil). It also means eating less animal and fish flesh, which is farther removed from those primary sources of energy. Animals and fish must eat plants or other fish or animals to get their nutrition, and the potency of the prana attenuates the farther away you get from those sources.

Here are several other reasons meat is not as pranically rich as other foods. First, it's often physically dirty. While we've seen progress over the last several decades in improving the living conditions of animals raised for human consumption, many still are not raised or slaughtered in a sanitary environment, which has obvious implications for cleanliness. Second, meat is often chemically dirty. Livestock and fowl raised for consumption at most large-scale farming operations, which supply the majority of our meat, are given sizeable quantities of hormones to ensure that they grow quickly, as well as significant doses of antibiotics to prevent diseases in their crowded conditions. These chemicals may help the farms that raise the chickens and cows and other animals produce more food more quickly, but they also reduce the purity of the prana in the food because they contain too many artificial additives. Third, meat is frequently emotionally dirty because the animals do experience great fear as they get closer to slaughter, and that negative emotion is embedded in both the animal's energy anatomy and physical tissues. Thus, when we eat meat, we are getting prana that is several levels removed from the purest sources of prana—it is second- or even third-hand energy—as well as physically, chemically, and emotionally dirty. (Note: Our suggestion to reduce meat consumption is not prompted by any political beliefs or personal judgments about the appropriateness of eating animals. This recommendation is made purely for the purpose of keeping your personal energy clean.)

Here are some simple dietary recommendations that will help you maintain a higher level of energetic cleanliness. Follow them to the extent that you feel comfortable.

- Let the bulk of your diet (at least 70 to 80 percent) consist of light, prana-intensive foods such as raw or lightly cooked vegetables, fresh fruits, and whole grains.
- If you can't or don't want to stop eating meat, at least limit your consumption a bit.
- Avoid pork, catfish, eel, and carp altogether. Pigs eat indiscriminately; catfish, eel, and carp are bottom-feeding fish. These are the absolute dirtiest foods you can eat.
- Scanning reveals that organic and natural foods or supplements contain more prana and prana of a higher quality than highly processed, preserved, or genetically modified foods. Thus, opt for clean, unprocessed foods when you can.
- Since excessive heat diminishes prana—it has the same effect on prana that it does on the vitamins and minerals in food—don't cook your food any longer than necessary.
- Try to use your microwave less. While microwaving is very convenient, prana is delicate, and clairvoyant observation and scanning indicate that microwaving greatly diminishes the amount of energy in your food.
- Since alcohol does have inherent cleansing properties, it's not all bad for you and your energy. So an occasional glass of wine or a beer is fine. Hard liquor, however, contains too much alcohol and has a negative effect on the body's prana.

To summarize, fruits, grains, and vegetables are the energetically cleanest foods. Next cleanest would be saltwater fish with scales; then, in order of declining cleanliness: saltwater fish without scales (such as shrimp), freshwater fish, fowl, and then land animals (red meat). The energetically dirtiest foods of all are pork and bottom-feeding fish, such as catfish, eel, and carp.

CUTTING CORDS

In the Hawaiian mystical tradition of Huna, which Grandmaster Choa studied extensively, it is taught that once thoughts are generated in the mind, they then attach themselves to the object contemplated via a thread of a sticky energetic substance called *aka*. Thus, you create an "aka thread" each time you think about, put your attention on, or have a reaction to something—a book you're reading, your children, preparing a meal, a hobby, or any other idle thought you may have. This thread or cord is evidence that you are directing your attention or personal energy toward an object. It's the same concept explained by the Chinese saying noted earlier, "The chi follows the yi." In Pranic Healing and Arhatic Yoga, we simply say that you are extending a portion of your aura to the object of your attention in the form of a thin strand of prana called an *energetic cord*. And the stronger our emotional connection to the person, issue, or object of attention—either positive or negative—the stronger and more tenacious the cord.

Cords are an energetic fact of life, and they can attach at any point or chakra in your aura. Their attachment points are fairly logical. If you're focused on reviewing a balance sheet for your business, an intellectual task, that cord might attach at the ajna, the chakra that governs conscious thought and deliberation. A cord for your children might attach at the front heart chakra, for love. If you have strong physical desire for someone, that cord might attach at the sex chakra. But the chakras that have the most cords attached to them are the front and back solar plexus chakras, because these chakras control the emotions in general.

Cords can be beneficial and productive, or harmful and nonproductive. They can also simply be neutral. As noted above, for people we love—our children or spouses, for example—we have strong cords that typically attach at the heart. Other good cords may attach us to warm memories or experiences, usually at the heart and/or solar plexus. Beneficial cords give us energetic sustenance. On the other hand, cords that connect us to a person we don't like or a circumstance that causes worry, fear, anxiety, or anger are a prime source of energetic contamination. Harmful cords can lead to energetic depletion or congestion. Neutral cords attach us to routine or mundane tasks or thoughts and cause neither benefit nor harm. For instance, if you're thinking about what to have for dinner, the thought might create a cord in your aura, perhaps from your ajna (conscious thought) to a magazine in which you read a recipe.

The intensity of the thought or emotion behind the thought determines both the size and strength of the cord. Most routine cords appear to clairvoyant observation as bundles of fine threads—very thin, bright strands, similar to the filament in a light bulb—extending outward from a person's aura. However, the appearance of cords also has an energetic logic. For instance, the cord between two people having a heated argument might be larger in diameter and grayish (dirty energy) with tinges of red (anger energy), while the cord between a mother and her child—a very strong bond—might appear to be almost a solid line, perhaps with light gold or pink (love energy) in it.

The goal in cord cutting is to eliminate the harmful influence of negative cords while leaving intact the beneficial influence of positive cords. Here is how you do it.

Exercise 4.1 **Cutting Cords**

The process of cutting negative cords is simple, but the positive effect on your aura and feelings of well-being can be rapid and dramatic. (Refer to figure 4.1 for the sequence of movements.)

1. Stand in a relaxed posture and take a couple of pranic breaths.

2. Put one hand above your head and slightly in front of your body with the palm facing downward. Put the other hand in front of your groin and slightly in front of your body with the palm facing up. Imagine you're holding a giant ball in front of your body (see the first position in figure 4.1).

3. Now move your hands slowly but firmly toward each other, both sweeping across the front of your body. As you do this, visualize that you are gathering all the negative cords attached to your chakras and your aura into a tight bundle in front of you. Establish your clear intent by saying to yourself silently something like, "I am now gathering together all the negative and nonproductive cords attached to my aura, and I will cut them completely."

4. Pull this tightened bunch of cords together in front of your front solar plexus chakra and imagine that you're holding them tightly in your bottom hand (see the second position in figure 4.1). (Many people can actually feel a bundle of cords as their hands get closer. If you can't feel them, just imagine them.)

5. As you hold the bundle in your bottom hand, slice through the cords three times sharply with your upper hand. Make the cut all the way through and

keep the cut close to your body (see the third position in figure 4.1). (Some people imagine that the bottom edge of their hand is a knife blade. Some students actually have a sharp knife that they keep only for cutting cords.) After you cut the cords, simply throw them into a wastebasket.

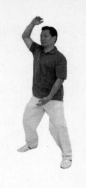

6. Next, you need to cut the cords attached to the back of your aura. So, visualize a picture of your back. Some people visualize the picture as half the size of real-life to make it easier.

7. Establish your clear intent to cut the negative cords attached to the back of your aura by repeating a phrase similar to the one you used to cut the cords in the front of your aura.

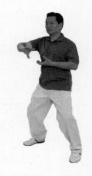

8. Position your hands so that one is above and the other below the visualized representation of yourself. It doesn't make any difference whether the right or left hand is above or below.

9. Then, as you did with the front cords, sweep your hands toward each other, gathering them into a bundle near your visualized back solar plexus chakra. Cut them three times with the same knife-hand motion, and throw the cords into a wastebasket.

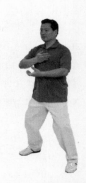

You can cut cords at any time and to any person, project, or object that causes you anxiety or fear. You can't overdo cord cutting or harm yourself in any way if you somehow don't do it perfectly. But it's easy to do. Simply visualize

Figure 4.1 **Cutting Cords**

the situation in front of you and a cord running from you to the triggering event, circumstance, or person. Most often cords of this type will attach at the front or back solar plexus, so it may help to visualize it attaching at one of these locations. Firmly and clearly establish your intent, then vigorously cut the cords three times as indicated. You should feel a sense of relaxation and tension relief very quickly after doing this.

THE CLEANSING POWER OF SALT

You may not know this, but salt—common table salt—was once considered a spice and food preservative of great value. It was often regarded as indispensable in sacrifices to harvest and fertility gods during ancient times, and Roman soldiers received part of their pay in salt. (Our English word *salary* is derived from the Latin *salarium,* which was that portion of the soldiers' compensation they received in salt. Eventually, *salarium*—and later, *salary*—became the general term for pay received for services rendered.)

Salt also has long been used in religious rituals, not only because of its value, but also for its ability as a cleansing agent. It is thus used, for instance, in many baptism rituals to symbolize the cleansing of a newborn as the baby is formally initiated into the church.

While today we know salt as among the most common and inexpensive of spices, it isn't widely known that there is a true energetic basis for its cleansing ability. Salt has the powerful ability to break up dirty and congested prana. A clairvoyant looking at salt sees that it is filled with highly concentrated green prana, which is among the most powerful colored pranas for breaking down and dissolving energetic blockages. It is for this reason that you can use salt to remove dirty energy from your aura as part of your own personal Energetic Hygiene program.

Exercise 4.2 **A Saltwater Bath**

You can enjoy the tremendous cleansing benefits of salt simply and easily while also taking advantage of another activity long cited for its ability to promote relaxation: a warm bath. Here's how to combine them both into one soothing—yet energizing—treat:

1. Pour one or two 26-ounce containers of table salt into a bathtub full of water. Warm water is usually better because it's physically relaxing, but it can be as hot or cold as you like. The water temperature will have no effect on the technique's cleansing ability. The salt can be iodized or not, but don't use Epsom salts. Epsom salts don't have the same energetic cleansing capability as table salt.

2. Sit in the bath for up to thirty minutes. Try to position yourself so that all your front body chakras—throat, front heart, front solar plexus, navel, and sex—are completely covered by the saltwater (depending on how tall you are and how big your tub is). Your back chakras will be cleansed regardless of your height or the tub size.

When you are done, wash off in the shower with soap, shampoo, or whatever other bath or shower gels you use.

After your saltwater bath, you will feel remarkably cleansed, refreshed, and relaxed. In fact, a clairvoyant observing someone taking a salt bath sees the body "smoking," as if fumes were coming out of it. This is the dirty energy leaving the aura. One interesting side effect of saltwater baths that most people find positive is an increase in sexual desire. That's because a saltwater bath thoroughly cleanses the lower body chakras that regulate sexual impulses and overall energy: the sex, basic, navel, and meng mein. These centers get contaminated very easily, especially if you spend a lot of time sitting or driving.

Most people find that taking a saltwater bath two or three times a week cleanses their energy body thoroughly. If you work in a heavily contaminated environment, or just need extra stress relief, you may want to take one more frequently.

For additional cleansing power, add up to ten drops of lavender oil. Lavender contains blue-violet prana, which enhances the green prana cleansing power of salt and is excellent for cleansing away dirty energy.

Exercise 4.3 **A Salt Shower**

There may be times when you're pressed for time or aren't able to use a bathtub. If so, here is how you can take a "salt shower":

1. Take a 26-ounce container of table salt with you into the shower. You can cut a hole in the original cardboard container, or pour it out into a more waterproof plastic tub or jar.

2. Pour a handful of salt into your palm and then rub it onto your body in a counterclockwise circular motion. Counterclockwise is the direction for cleansing during Pranic Healing, so rubbing the salt into your body in this way magnifies the salt's natural cleansing abilities. (Note on directional orientation: Imagine a clock on your body, facing outward.)

3. Focus on the organs and energy centers you can reach: liver, spleen, front and back spleen chakras, the navel and sex chakras, the front solar plexus chakra, the front heart and throat chakras. Most people can usually reach the basic and meng mein chakras, and if you can, rub some salt on the kidneys and adrenal glands as well. (Congratulations on your flexibility if you can reach your back solar

plexus and heart chakras!) Let the salt scrub stay on your body for several minutes; then wash it off. A salt shower doesn't cleanse you as thoroughly as a salt bath, but it can still be an effective Energetic Hygiene measure.

You can magnify the salt's cleansing ability by mixing the salt in a container with about ten to twenty drops of lavender oil.

Exercise 4.4 **A Cleansing Swim**

If you want to combine good Energetic Hygiene with your next vacation, or you happen to live on a coast, you can take advantage of the largest natural saltwater bath available, the ocean. Even though our oceans do contain more pollution than they should, still, the salt in seawater really has the power to clean away dirty energy. Here's how to do it:

1. Simply stand or swim in the ocean up to your neck for twenty or thirty minutes, and let the waves wash away your dirty energy.

2. Turn around several times to allow the wave motion to swirl around both your front and back chakras.

These three Energetic Hygiene techniques are simple and easy to integrate into your daily routine, but they are extremely helpful in ensuring that the prana in your aura stays fresh and clean.

PRACTICE UPDATE: ADDING ENERGETIC HYGIENE TO YOUR ROUTINE

You should try to take at least two saltwater baths per week. That will provide you with a minimum level of overall energetic cleanliness. If you are under a great deal of stress or work in an area of high contamination (for example, as a doctor or nurse in a hospital, as a law enforcement officer, or at any job in a city with excessive air pollution), you may want to take them more frequently.

Cord cutting should be employed regularly throughout the day. It's simple enough that it can be done at just about any time, and with practice, you can be fairly discreet. For instance, cut cords to all negative influences before meditation to keep your mind clear. Or perhaps you're going into a meeting at work with someone you don't get along with. Before the meeting, visualize that person and cut cords to him or her. If you're worried about freeway driving but have to make a long trip, simply cut cords to that fear. And, before you go to bed at night, you can help promote deeper and easier sleep by forming an intention to cut all nonproductive or negative cords, then physically cutting those cords. Just remember, you can cut cords to any fear- or anxiety-reducing event, person, or trigger.

Dietary changes are always a personal choice. But if you're serious about increasing your energy, you should try to reduce consumption of red meat and eliminate pork, catfish, and eel altogether. Try that for a month, and see how you feel. Quite likely, you'll feel your level of energy increase. And if you're so inclined, you can then make additional changes.

Chapter 5   The Cleansing Physical Exercises

Linda Tedrahn of Ohio performed the Nine Energizing Breaths for three consecutive days and felt the results immediately. "I know without a doubt that I had more energy," she says. "Each day I got up earlier and was able to stay up later. I immediately felt tons of energy. I loved it. I haven't been able to do any aerobic exercises due to my body condition, and this has given me hope. I know my heart and blood were circulating more than running a marathon. Thank you for sharing this with the world."

Have you ever wondered why you often feel energized after beginning or engaging in a regular exercise program? Think about it. You've expended energy to exercise, and yet you frequently feel *more* energized after you're done. There are several reasons for this. First, there's the primary physiological benefit of aerobic (endurance) and anaerobic (strength) training on the body, which is to build up your stamina and power. You are increasing the ability of your physical body to perform athletically at a higher level. Depending on the vigor and intensity of your training regimen, you're likely improving your hand-eye coordination, teaching your body to move more quickly or with more agility, getting your muscles and nervous system more in sync, building up your ability to run longer distances, and/or increasing the amount of weight you can lift. All these activities make your physical body stronger, faster, more powerful, more efficient—and more energetic. Second, there is evidence that exercise stimulates the production of natural proteins in the brain that produce many positive effects on your attitude and energy level, while inhibiting some of the proteins that produce harmful effects. For instance, numerous studies have shown that physical exercise increases the level of your endorphins, chemicals that are associated with pain regulation and the brain's so-called pleasure center. In one very interesting recent research effort, a team of investigators at Duke University found that three thirty-minute sessions of aerobic exercise per week were an "effective, robust treatment for patients with major depression." The study found that it increased patients' serotonin level (the same chemical affected by anti-depression medications) and decreased the level of adrenaline and cortisol (two hormones released during times of high stress and associated with the fight-or-flight response).[1] Another study indicated that even light activity such as walking can keep the mind sharp and reduce the likelihood of Alzheimer's disease and dementia by inhibiting the amount of a protein called amyloid, which in Alzheimer's patients clogs the brain and interferes with its messaging capacity.[2]

These are the empirical and the scientific reasons exercise boosts your energy and makes you feel less stressed: it increases your body's ability to perform physically, and it has a positive effect on your biochemistry.

There is also a very fundamental energetic reason exercise promotes vitality and relieves tension: physical exercise—stretching, running, jumping, aerobics, lifting weights, and even brisk walking—has a cleansing effect on the body's aura; it literally loosens and expels dirty and congested prana from your meridians and chakras. A clairvoyant can see dark stains in the aura of a person who is exercising becoming lighter to the point where the stains may even dissolve completely.

There are certain physical movements that are more effective than others at cleansing your aura. For instance, some yoga *asanas,* or postures, and many internal martial arts, such as tai chi chuan and chi kung, were developed specifically to cleanse and energize the aura. But these sorts of routines, while effective, often take time to learn and to practice. Some also demand strength or suppleness that not everyone is capable of. However, there is another way that you can use exercise to attain optimal Energetic Hygiene in a short amount of time and with minimal physical exertion. It's a mild set of stretches and twists taught in Pranic Healing and Arhatic Yoga called simply the Cleansing Physical Exercises. You can use them alone as they are presented in this chapter, or as an adjunct or warm-up to your regular exercise routine. They're easy to learn and perform, but they're extremely powerful.

There are three reasons the Cleansing Physical Exercises are so effective:

1. **They create a focused "pumping effect" on the chakras.** Each movement in the Cleansing Physical Exercises has a pumping effect on the part of the body being exercised. This results in an associated opening and closing of the body's chakras and meridians in that area. As the chakras and meridians open and close, they break up and eject dirty or congested prana.

2. **They lightly energize the chakras before cleaning them.** This is one of the real secrets of the Cleansing Physical Exercises and many of the other teachings of Pranic Healing and Arhatic Yoga. For those body parts where you can do this in the Cleansing Physical Exercises, you begin with a *clockwise* motion to slightly energize the area and then follow that with a *counterclockwise* motion to clean it. (In Pranic Healing, students learn that a counterclockwise hand motion will manually clean a dirty area of the aura, and a clockwise motion can be used to energize it. It's the same principle used in acupuncture when needles are twisted back and forth, or even in putting in a screw: twist clockwise to drive it in, and counterclockwise to take it out. However, a more advanced technique for rapid cleansing is to lightly energize an area in order to loosen up the dirty energy so that it can be cleaned out more easily.)

3. **They use a logical cleaning sequence.** The exercises are performed in a head-to-toe-sequence in order to drive the dirty energy down through the body and then flush it out through the feet. This ensures that the more delicate energetic areas—the chakras of the upper body and head—are clean.

Because the Cleansing Physical Exercises warm up the physical body as well as cleanse the energy body, they are good to perform just before the Nine Energizing Breaths. In Arhatic Yoga, students are advised to perform them both before and after meditation. Prior to meditation, as you have read here, they expel dirty energy and prepare the body to receive fresh, clean prana. After meditation, their strong cleansing action disperses the prana that can settle in the aura as energetic congestion after sitting quietly in meditation for a period of time.

The simple, gentle movements of the Cleansing Physical Exercises were designed to be performed by anyone—regardless of fitness level. However, there are two things you should keep in mind so that you can perform them safely and effectively. First, if you have any doubts at all about your ability or fitness to perform this routine, get the advice of your physician. Second, keep your movements smooth and fluid. There should be no strain at any time. Never "stretch into pain"—that is, don't make any movement that takes you beyond a comfortable stretch into an ache. Put another way, you should hurt neither during nor after these movements.

Exercise 5.1 **The Cleansing Physical Exercises**

The Cleansing Physical Exercises are brief enough so that most people can complete two entire sets in less than five minutes. Perform the entire routine just as you see it here, in the order presented. To take an exercise out of sequence won't disrupt their purifying ability, but they're designed to clean from head to toe, in order to flush the dirty energy from the more delicate areas (head) and chakras (crown, ajna, throat, heart) through the less delicate lower chakras (basic, sex) and then out the feet. It's just a more efficient way of quickly cleaning the energy body that doesn't leave any energetic congestion in more sensitive areas. However, if you have some physical limitation that prevents you from doing one or another exercise, either skip it or do the best you can with it and move on to the exercises you can perform.

1. **Eye rotations.** While keeping your head and neck still, roll your eyes twelve times clockwise, then twelve times counterclockwise. (Use the same directional orientation as mentioned with regard to the salt shower: imagine a clock on your body, facing outward.) Sometimes a perfect circle is difficult to achieve, so it may be easier to think about moving your eyes in four directions: beginning at twelve o'clock, to three o'clock, to six o'clock, to nine o'clock, and then back to twelve o'clock, for one clockwise revolution. Simply reverse for counterclockwise.

2. **Horizontal neck rotations.** Begin facing forward. Gently twist your head left and then right twelve times. As you rotate in each direction, presuming you have no physical restrictions, you should make a 90-degree turn left and right.

3. **Vertical neck rotations.** Begin with your head up and chin slightly back, facing forward. Smoothly pivot your head up and down twelve times. Remember, don't stretch into pain.

4. **Downward hand flings.** With your arms hanging at your sides and your hands open, pivot at the elbow and briskly pull your forearms up while balling your fists. Then quickly pivot at the elbow and fling your forearms down while opening your hands. Perform the up and down motion twelve times.

5. **Hand looseners.** Extend your arms straight out in front of you, with one palm down and one up. Open and close your hands quickly twelve times. Then reverse, putting the other palm down and the first one up and repeat the movement. (Those who have practiced any internal martial arts may recognize this as an exercise taught to open the *lao gong* points [they roughly correspond with the palm chakras] in the center of the hands. It increases your sensitivity to energy and allows your energy to be more easily transferred to an opponent during a fight.)

6. **Wrist rotations.** Extend your arms forward, palms facing down, fingers outstretched. Roll your wrists twelve times each in both directions.

7. **Shoulder rotations.** Stretch your arms out to the side horizontally, palms downward. Make circles with your arms moving backward twelve times. Then reverse the motion, and make twelve forward circles. Perform this at a moderate pace, not so slowly that you don't feel the shoulders stretch a bit, but not so fast that you feel a strain.

8. **Torso twist.** Extend your arms straight out from your sides so that they are parallel to the ground. With your feet about shoulder-width apart, twist twelve times to the right and to the left. As with the neck rotations, try to get your torso to a 90-degree twist, but don't strain. With each twist, allow your arms to sink down, so that they're at your sides as you conclude.

9. **Shoulder shrugs.** Drop your chin to your chest and shrug your shoulders slightly forward while allowing your arms to hang loosely in front of you. Breathe in while pulling your head and shoulders back as far as they can comfortably go. Then move your head and shoulders forward while exhaling. Do this twelve times.

10. **Hip rotations.** Put your hands on your hips and bend your knees slightly. Rotate your hips twelve times clockwise and then twelve times counterclockwise.

11. **Squats.** Bend slightly at the knees, and then perform quarter squats. See if you can do one hundred per session. Unlike a full squat, in which your buttocks touch your heels when you dip, with a quarter squat, you dip your knees only a little. Energetically, the quarter squat is only slightly less powerful than a full squat, and it's much easier on the knees. If you wish to do a deeper squat, feel free to do so. The squat charges your basic chakra, which is the principal chakra regulating your overall level of energy.

12. **Knee rotations.** With your legs together and knees slightly flexed, place your palms on your kneecaps and move your legs in circles. Rotate them twelve times clockwise and twelve times counterclockwise.

13. **Ankle rotations.** Balance yourself on your right leg, lift your left leg a few inches off the ground, and extend it slightly in front of you. As you did with your wrists, rotate your ankle twelve times clockwise and twelve times counterclockwise. Then repeat with the right ankle.

PRACTICE UPDATE: ADDING THE CLEANSING PHYSICAL EXERCISES TO YOUR ROUTINE

For optimum Energetic Hygiene, you should try to perform at least one set of the Cleansing Physical Exercises daily. If you have to break up your practice, get them in when you can. However, they work best in concert with some of the other exercises you're learning here. For example, it's very effective to perform them just before pranic breathing practice, the Nine Energizing Breaths, and/or meditation. If your daily routine permits you to meditate and perform the Nine Energizing Breaths, you can add the Cleansing Physical Exercises after meditation and just before the Nine Energizing Breaths to further prepare your body for the high-quality prana generated by the Nine Energizing Breaths.

Part Three

The Nine Energizing Breaths

Chapter 6   Performing the Nine Energizing Breaths

I gauge how much energy I have based on how much and how intensely I can exercise. I like to go on long bike rides through the hills of the area where I live in Southern California. After doing the Nine Energizing Breaths for a few days, I noticed that my bicycle rides became very easy; my diaphragm and chest wall muscles were relaxed, making deep breathing effortless. The rest of the muscles in my body felt relaxed yet vitalized. In fact, on the day of this writing, I went on a long bike ride up a two-mile steep hill, something I never thought I'd be able to do in my lifetime, and did it with surprising ease, a fast recovery, and an upbeat, energized (not depleted) feeling the rest of the day once I was done. I also notice that my brain seems to be getting the benefit of the energy flow through the nervous system, with better visual acuity, and memory, and yet an emotional calm.

ERIC B. ROBINS, MD

It has long been the practice in spiritual traditions, both Eastern and Western, to withhold the most advanced wisdom and most powerful techniques from all but a small group of initiates. This was often done by presenting these inner teachings, as they are often called, only through word of mouth. When these teachings were written down—and even when they were presented orally—the deeper and more advanced wisdom was often obscured through the use of metaphors, stories, or parables. For example, the lotus flowers that appear in Sanskrit texts are really part of the instructions for high-level meditation techniques. The steaming cauldron of Taoist yoga is a symbol for the development of internal power or chi. And the parables of Jesus are thought by many to contain not only guidance for salvation in the traditional Christian sense but also mystical teachings akin to those of Buddhist, Kabbalistic, or Taoist masters. In this way, ancient esoteric knowledge was passed down through the ages from the teacher to only the most adept students, for only these initiates would pick up on the true inner meaning of the teachings. The Nine Energizing Breaths are part of that ancient esoteric knowledge.

HISTORY OF THE NINE ENERGIZING BREATHS

Though they are reported to have been introduced to the West by Edwin J. Dingle, a British explorer and journalist who traveled throughout China and Tibet in the early part of the twentieth century, the Nine Energizing Breaths are actually Indian in origin. Guru Padmasambhava,[1] more popularly known as Guru Rinpoche, was an Indian Buddhist teacher from what was then Udyan—now Swat in Kashmir, Pakistan—an area renowned for its powerful spiritual mystics.[2] Padmasambhava traveled to Tibet in 747 AD at the invitation of King Thi-srong-detsan and began teaching Tantric Buddhism. Also known as Vajrayana (Sanskrit for "vehicle of the diamond or thunderbolt"), Tantric Buddhism is characterized by teachings that cut through ignorance "like a thunderbolt" or "diamond." The diamond also stands for that which is permanent, unchanging, and unbreakable in reality and in man versus the illusion of the world around us.[3] It was in the course of his Tantric Buddhist instruction that Padmasambhava revealed many of the ancient yogic techniques and ideas that were the basis of the Nine Energizing Breaths.

During his travels throughout Asia, Dingle eventually was charged to take over a newspaper in Singapore called the *Strait Times*.[4] While there, he met an unassuming individual who was actually a formidable spiritual teacher called the Sage of Singapore. One evening this man invited Dingle to a nearby temple to witness an important ceremony that turned out to be a life-transforming experience for the young writer. At the temple, Dingle saw the sage wearing very little clothing and performing what he found out later was yogic breathing. An attendant stoked a fire that was heating two iron sandals until they were red hot. The sage placed his feet into the sandals and started walking around. After the sandals were removed, the sage's feet were unmarked. Dingle, quite naturally, was unsure of what he had just seen. Thinking that perhaps he had been hypnotized, he touched the red hot sandals with his fingers and was badly burned and scarred.

Dingle's later travels took him to Burma, where he had another auspicious encounter with the sage. One evening, as he lay on a chair on the balcony of his bungalow, he heard footsteps on the stairs. In the moonlight, he saw the outline of a man and heard a voice he recognized. It was the sage, who said only, "Brother, they are waiting for you in Tibet," before quickly departing into the night.

Shortly thereafter, Dingle left for Tibet, and after a long and difficult trip, during which he suffered attacks by wild animals and robbers, as well as a bout with malaria, he finally arrived. He met up with his teacher and quickly became his apprentice. It took a while for Dingle to make sense of the things he saw in Tibet and the instruction he received in spirituality, meditation, and breathing, but in time, he learned the exercises that he later brought to the West and taught through his Institute of Mentalphysics, which he founded in 1927. Included among these teachings was an early version of the Nine Energizing Breaths.

The Nine Energizing Breaths are also part of what are called esoteric *root teachings,* the truths and techniques that are common to all spiritual systems throughout the history of the world. As a spiritual teacher with a long and broad lineage and ready access to these root teachings, Grandmaster Choa Kok Sui adapted, enhanced, and reintroduced the Nine Energizing Breaths into his Pranic Healing and Arhatic Yoga classes about fifteen years ago. As mentioned, they are exercises of extraordinary power and simplicity, and they are presented here without any metaphorical trappings. In fact, they are stripped down to their essence, which is why they're so simple to learn.

However, do not mistake simplicity for lack of sophistication or effectiveness. They *will* energize you!

THE ORIGINAL VERSUS THE ENHANCED EXERCISES

The Tibetan breathing exercises taught by Edwin Dingle through his Mentalphysics organization are undeniably powerful. After all, that's the routine that enabled Laura Appelgren to defeat cancer, and thousands of others to dramatically improve their lives. But they're also quite lengthy. Dingle's students were instructed to work up to performing the seven main exercises—three through nine—seven times each, and to build up to holding their breath for sixty seconds for each repetition of those seven exercises. This means the full routine would take nearly an hour. If you wish to perform the original routine, feel free to do so.[5] They're still available in various forms from the Institute of Mentalphysics (see Further

Reading). Most students feel, though, that the modified version, offered here as the Nine Energizing Breaths, is more powerful and certainly more convenient, as it takes much less time.

Here is a summary of Grandmaster Choa's three major enhancements to the exercises:[6]

1. **Placing the tip of the tongue on the roof of the mouth just behind the hard palate and holding it there during the entire routine (except for one small portion of the Second Energizing Breath).** This modification greatly facilitates the flow of prana through the body by connecting the circuit between the two largest energy channels of the body, one running down the front and the other up the back. Those familiar with acupuncture or such Taoist meditations as the "microcosmic orbit," "small heavenly circle," or "warm current meditation" may recognize these channels as the functional or conception meridian (front) and the governor meridian (back).

2. **Changing the breathing rhythm for the first two Energizing Breaths.** In the modified version, you perform the same total number of breaths as Dingle's original routine for the first two exercises, but employ a different breathing rhythm that generates more energy. You'll read about the details in the specific instructions for each of the exercises.

3. **Contracting and holding your pubococcygeal or PC muscles during the third through the ninth Energizing Breath.** The PC muscles control your bowel and urinary functions. When you contract the PC muscle group, it is as if you are trying to prevent yourself from going to the bathroom, both front and back. When you contract the PC muscles during these exercises, it pushes the prana from the lower chakras to the upper chakras and also out into your extremities. For women, the front portion of this movement is the same as Kegel exercises. For practitioners of yoga, this is a type of *bandha* (see sidebar). This contraction is the modification that dramatically increases the power of the Nine Energizing Breaths while significantly shortening the time required to perform them.

Bandha and PC Contraction

Bandha is a Sanskrit word meaning "lock" or "tighten." It is a physical tightening of a portion of the body, held for a period of time during the practice of the asanas or pranayama. A bandha locks in the prana and then guides it into the *sushumna nadi*, or the large energy channel running up the spine from its base to the head, where it is then used for spiritual development and enlightenment. Depending on the yogic source material and style of yoga, there are generally three types of band-has—*jalandhara* (*jala* means "net"), *uddiyana* ("fly up") and *mula*, ("root" or "base"), and then a fourth, *maha*, ("great"), which is the simultaneous application of the other three bandhas. The jalandhara bandha is a lock of the chin into the notch in the front of the throat. The uddiyana bandha involves an exaggerated pulling in and up of the stomach and diaphragm after a full exhalation. The mula bandha is described in some yoga texts and training exactly as the PC contraction is detailed here. Others teach that it is a contraction of only the back half of the PC area, or just the perineum and the anus. In either case, it is a powerful lock that pushes the strong physical energy of the lower chakras throughout the rest of the body. The PC contraction supercharges the Nine Energizing Breaths.

EFFECT OF THE NINE ENERGIZING BREATHS ON YOUR ENERGETIC ANATOMY

When we say that the Nine Energizing Breaths "increase your energy," it isn't a vague promise that you'll feel like you just had a double espresso; it's a veri-fiable energetic fact. The Nine Energizing Breaths produce the same effect on your energetic anatomy that physical exercise produces on your body: it makes it bigger and more "muscular." Clairvoyants observing those practic-ing the Nine Energizing Breaths report that the overall aura increases in size, brightness, and strength and that the chakras bulge outward and become more dynamic, which means they spin more smoothly and rapidly.

As with physical exercise and the body, this growth of the aura is temporary initially, and the aura and chakras eventually shrink back to their prior size. But with regular practice, the aura and chakras become energetically conditioned, and they continue to grow and get bigger and stronger as long as you con-tinue the routine—again, just as the physical body responds to regular physical exercise. In fact, performing the Nine Energizing Breaths in the specific pre-scribed sequence produces what is referred to in Arhatic Yoga as an "energetic compounding effect," which means that the energy generated each day builds upon the previous day's efforts. In time, your energetic anatomy becomes—and stays—larger, stronger, denser, and brighter. Both the quantity and quality of your personal energy dramatically increase, and you can feel the difference.

In addition to this general effect on the energetic anatomy, each exercise in the Nine Energizing Breaths also produces a specific effect on each individual chakra, certain sets of chakras, and different areas of the body. For instance, the First Energizing Breath cleanses, charges, and balances the energy in your head and on the right and left side of your body, while the Second Energizing Breath cleanses the energy along your main back meridian, the chakras along your back (basic, meng mein, back solar plexus, and back heart), and spinal column.

THE NINE ENERGIZING BREATHS AND ENERGY, REJUVENATION, YOUTHFULNESS, AND LONGEVITY

Judging by the countless cosmetics used to make us appear younger, the growing number of drugs to enhance libido, and the variety of surgical procedures to lift, peel, augment, or suction this or that part of the body, our contemporary world certainly has a fixation on youthfulness and longevity. While modern medical science may enable the body to *appear* younger, the Nine Energizing Breaths, based on energetic truths about the way the body produces and absorbs prana, can actually help your body *be* more youthful and rejuvenated. And unlike current medical, cosmetic, or pharmaceutical solutions, this "true way of energy," as it might be called, is safe, simple, inexpensive, quick, and effective.

Working on both the physical and energetic level, the Nine Energizing Breaths deliver a range of powerful benefits, including the following:

- cleaner, stronger chakras
- stronger organs and a more robust immune system
- enhanced healing ability, of both self and others
- greater absorption of energy to promote youthfulness and rejuvenation of the body, as well as longevity

Cleaner, Stronger Chakras; Stronger Organs and Immune System

As you read in chapter 5, "Cleansing Physical Exercises," when you alternately tense and relax the muscles, you initiate a pumping effect that promotes pranic respiration. This helps the chakras expel dirty energy and draw in clean, fresh prana, which strengthens the body and the organs.

However, when you perform the Nine Revitalizing Breaths, you not only tense your muscles and put your tongue on your palate, you also hold your breath using powerful rhythm and retention techniques, perform a range of dynamic movements, and squeeze the PC muscle. These actions make the cleansing effect of the exercise exponentially more powerful. Thus, the flow of prana through the chakras and organs is greatly accelerated, and the chakras are synchronized, which helps you not only to become gently energized but also to remain calm as you increase your energy. It helps charge up your entire immune system and provide preventive health maintenance for your energy body.

Enhanced Healing Ability

Many energy healing systems teach practitioners to generate prana or chi in their bodies and then project it into the patient. Most chi kung healing systems, for instance, teach students to build up a surplus of chi in their tan tien, or the energy storage area under the navel chakra, and use that energy for healing. The drawback is that, since the healers are ultimately using their own energy, their own personal stores of energy will be used up. One of the big advantages of the Pranic Healing system is that healers learn to draw in healing energy through one chakra and project it through another (the palm chakra); they don't use their own energy. As a result, they are not as prone to energetic depletion as other healers. However, even without using much of their own energy, pranic healers can still become tired or mentally fatigued. Pranic healers who consistently practice the Nine Energizing Breaths, though, report that they help shore up their personal energy supplies; they don't get as tired when working on a variety of clients. As a result, they're more effective healers. The experience of pranic healer Kei Okubo from Riverside, California, is typical. "I used to have shoulder pain after doing deep tissue massage on clients," she says. "However, since about 2003, I have been doing a set of the Nine Energizing Breaths between clients and have not had shoulder pain since. And I have been regularly practicing the Nine Energizing Breaths right after meditation for about the past year. They have facilitated amazing healing results for my clients and reduced their healing session time by approximately half."

Rejuvenation and Youthfulness

We've all seen people in their seventies with the drive and energy of someone decades younger. And we all probably know someone in their twenties who is frequently tired or doesn't have the energy you would expect someone that age to have. How can one person have vigor well into advanced age and another, much younger, be chronically tired or listless? Medical science or psychology may not have a definitive response, but there is an energetic answer in your aura: youthfulness is determined not by your chronological age but by the dynamism of your chakras, their ability to spin smoothly and quickly, both clockwise and counterclockwise.

Children, literally the most youthful of us, have the most dynamic chakras, as determined by clairvoyant observation. The chakras of children spin rapidly. Not coincidentally, children have seemingly boundless energy, and they heal rapidly.

However, as we get older, the stresses of life wear on us and wear our body down. We allow ourselves to become energetically contaminated. Our chakras become dirtier and spin less quickly and smoothly. The prana exchange becomes less efficient. The chakras gradually lose their ability to absorb fresh prana and expel dirty or used-up prana. The organs controlled by each chakra receive less fresh prana, and organ function begins to diminish. As a result of this energetic slowdown, the outward signs of what we call the "aging process" become evident. We tire more easily. Our sex drive isn't what it used to be. The skin loses its glow, the muscles lose their tone, the immune system doesn't protect us as well as it used to, and we don't bounce back as quickly from health problems.

Physical exercise will help slow down the aging process because, as you have read, it provides a workout not only to the muscles but also to the chakras. However, to truly reclaim youthfulness, to rejuvenate the body, you need to perform specially designed exercises that not only work out the body but also draw in prana and "physicalize" it, or actually instill it into the tissues of the body. With its unique blend of breath retention, muscle tension, and modifications that highly activate the body's energy pathways, the Nine Energizing Breaths do just that. They drive prana deep into the muscles, bones, organs, and connective tissue to strengthen and tone the physical body. The chakras are substantially cleansed, and they regain their spin and dynamism. The characteristics of physical aging begin to be reversed, and the body truly regains youthfulness. The improvement can be quite noticeable, as Southern California medical sales manager Anthony Guidera relates. "I am in an operating room almost every day, so I need to stay mentally sharp, and I need my energy level to be consistently high," he says. "The Nine Energizing Breaths have not only doubled my energy level, they've calmed my emotions. On top of that, it seems like they've also slowed down the physical aging process. I will be fifty in September, and when people ask me my age and I tell them, they look shocked and say, 'You look like you're in your thirties.'"

The Secret of Longevity: The Nine Energizing Breaths and Meditation

We've all heard enough stories of the holy man or "mountain-top guru" that it's almost a cliché: the long hair and beard, the robe, the ascetic diet, the isolation, the hours of meditation in a lotus position, and the whispers that he's actually hundreds of years old.

As with many aspects of the spiritual or esoteric life—even those aspects that have become legends—there is often some truth behind the stories, and in this case, it has to do with meditation and how it can be used to support longevity.

Certain meditations, properly done, will draw down the highest grade of prana, called *divine spiritual energy,* through your crown and into your aura. Even mild meditations such as simple breath awareness or mindfulness routines will often enable you to calm the mind sufficiently so that you can unconsciously make contact with a higher power, through which you gain access to this powerful cleansing energy. This higher power goes by different names in different systems: higher self, Christ Consciousness, inner teacher, and many others. In Pranic Healing and Arhatic Yoga, we refer to it as the Higher Soul.

This energy enters into your aura from your Higher Soul through your spiritual cord, which is a thin thread running between your crown chakra and your Higher Soul. When this contact takes place and the downward energy flow occurs, many powerful and positive changes can happen, ranging from mental calmness to physical healing to inner peace to enlightenment. At a minimum, the energy will circulate around and through your aura and help dissipate the contamination you pick up during daily life, providing a kind of automatic Energetic Hygiene effect. However—and this is very important—only a minimal amount of this meditation-generated prana will enter the physical body, and for the physical body to be rejuvenated for longer life, it needs to have a great quantity of this divine spiritual energy infused into the muscles, bones, organs, and tissues.

That's what the pulsing action of the Nine Energizing Breaths does when you perform the routine immediately following meditation. When you inhale and tense your muscles, you "stuff" the spiritual meditation energy that's floating around in your aura, along with the more "physical" energy produced by the Nine Energizing Breaths, deep into the body's tissues. Then, when you vigorously exhale, you expel dirty energy from the physical body. Driving both high-quality divine spiritual energy and the more physical Nine Energizing Breaths energy deep into the muscles, organs, and bones while expelling dirty energy is the true secret of physical rejuvenation and actual longevity.

Certain tai chi chuan and yoga routines may also add years to your life, but in a much more gradual and less dynamic way because most don't quickly and safely generate the raw energy that the Nine Energizing Breaths does.

Traditional Esoteric Exercises for Youthfulness and Rejuvenation Are Much More Complex

Esoteric literature is filled with exercises, techniques, and meditations designed to generate energy for youthfulness and longevity. The Taoists have one of the most well-known and well-preserved bodies of work devoted to rejuvenation. However, to read some of their instructions today, it is clear this is a routine designed for the lifestyle of a reclusive monk, for it is an almost around-the-clock endeavor. Certainly, it would require a commitment far beyond the time required to perform the Nine Energizing Breaths. Traditional Taoist teachings include a regimen that incorporated lengthy meditations and breathing exercises, plus regular—almost hourly—massages with hands, stones, or balls and tapping the body with sticks, bundles of sticks, and even metal rods. The idea was to generate the energy and then manually "pack" the energy into the tissues with massages and hitting. The two most commonly known techniques you may read about today, often called the tendon-changing and bone-marrow-washing exercises, are derived from this tradition.

Another common rejuvenation practice in Taoism, Hinduism, and many forms of yoga is retention of sex energy. Though today many read texts on Taoist sexual practices or Tantric yoga, and books such as the *Kama Sutra*, as simple aids to pleasure, they are actually how-to books on cultivating sexual energy for spiritual enlightenment. The idea is that the sex act is sacred and that sexual energy, when properly cultivated, can be "spiritual gasoline." However, the key is "properly cultivated," for many of these books greatly simplify what can be a difficult and/or dangerous process. Like kundalini, sexual energy can be very powerful and should be developed only under the direction of an experienced teacher.

The movements and PC lock of the Nine Energizing Breaths enable you to gently and safely exercise the main chakras governing sexual energy—the basic, sex, and navel chakras—so that you get both physical benefits (stronger, more pleasurable intercourse and more sustained sex drive), as well energetic benefits (more physical vigor and vitality). And you get both without the time-consuming practice required by the traditional methods or the danger of possibly allowing the sexual energy to be developed without sufficient control.

Table 6.1 provides a summary of the Nine Energizing Breaths, their names, and the chakras and body parts each exercise energizes.

TABLE 6.1 EFFECTS OF THE NINE ENERGIZING BREATHS

ENERGIZING BREATH	ENERGETIC EFFECT ON THE AURA AND BODY
First Energizing Breath	This exercise cleans and balances the energy on both sides of the brain and on the left and right sides of the body. The body's entire energy level is balanced and harmonized. Thus, this exercise is called Balancing Breathing in some systems. You may also see it referred to in other literature as Caduceus Breathing, because it causes the energy to flow up through the body in a spiral fashion, through the *ida* (yin) and *pingala* (yang) channels that wrap around the sushumna, or central channel. In fact, clairvoyant observation shows that the First Energizing Breath performed alone can increase the aura's size up to 300 percent; however, the effect is temporary.
Second Energizing Breath	This exercise cleans and balances the energy in the head, neck, and spine, as well as the major meridians running through those areas. It is good for mental work and increasing mental efficiency. It is also known as Rapid Turtle Breathing in some systems.
Third Energizing Breath	This exercise pushes energy throughout the entire body, especially from the lower to the upper chakras.

TABLE 6.1 **THE EFFECT OF THE NINE ENERGIZING BREATHS...(continued)**

Fourth Energizing Breath	This exercise circulates energy throughout the entire body. It cleans the front and back heart chakra, as well as the upper back and chest.
Fifth Energizing Breath	This exercise cleans and energizes the upper chakras; especially the front and back spleen and heart chakras, and the throat chakra. The practitioner will sometimes feel a "melting" sensation as the chakras are charged.
Sixth Energizing Breath	Physically, this exercise loosens up the shoulders and neck. Energetically, it has a strong stress reduction effect because it expels dirty energy from the front and back solar plexus chakras.
Seventh Energizing Breath	Physically, this exercise loosens up the shoulders and neck and is very good for massage therapists or anyone else who uses their upper back or shoulders. Energetically, it cleans and energizes the back solar plexus, meng mein, and basic chakras, as well as the lower lumbar region of the spine.
Eighth Energizing Breath	This exercise has a strong cleansing, energizing, and regenerating effect on the entire body, and especially the organs of the trunk, the head, and the brain. It helps activate key pranic "pumping stations" in the meng mein and back of the neck that move the prana from the lower to the upper chakras. It also cleans and regulates the sex and throat chakras, which are connected energetically. As a result, this exercise will help regulate and normalize the sex drive. If your sex drive is low, it will be boosted. If it's high, it will become more balanced.
Ninth Energizing Breath	This exercise cleans, balances, and regulates both sides of the body, the entire aura, and all the chakras. It is particularly beneficial for people who sit for extended periods of time.

PRACTICING THE NINE ENERGIZING BREATHS

The Nine Energizing Breaths are fairly easy to perform, but as with any new physical movement routine, it takes a bit of practice before you can coordinate the breathing, the PC lock, and the arm and leg positions smoothly. Most people have the movements mastered within a week or two of daily practice.

One of the first questions beginners ask is how many times they should perform each of the exercises and how often. The routine will enable you to build up quite a bit of energy and improve your general vigor in a surprisingly little amount of time, so it is advisable to not exceed the recommendations. Otherwise, excess energy could build up and create discomfort. Here is the recommended practice schedule for beginners:

- **First Energizing Breath**. Do one set, which is 7 breaths through each nostril.
- **Second Energizing Breath**. Do one set, which is 49 rapid breaths according to the indicated rhythm.
- **Third through Ninth Energizing Breath**. One repetition each. Hold breath and PC contraction on the Third Energizing Breath for five seconds only. Hold breath and PC contraction on the Fourth through Ninth Energizing Breath only through the end of the physical movement and no longer.

The above sequence constitutes one set of the Nine Energizing Breaths, and you can perform one such set daily. After a month, if you have no feelings of discomfort or being overenergized, you can practice a second set daily, and then once a week you can perform up to three sets.

Performing More Than One Set

Here is how you perform more than one set. Your second and third sets begin at the Third Energizing Breath; you don't repeat the First or Second Energizing Breath in subsequent sets of the entire routine. And you will perform two repetitions of each exercise in a row, rather than doing the Third through the Ninth one time, and then repeating the Third through the Ninth a second or third time. After you learn Pranic Healing, in which you are taught sweeping to clean away excess energy, you can increase the number of sets to three daily because you will then have the ability to clean your aura if you get overenergized.

Other Basic Practice Tips

Here are some other guidelines to help you optimize your performance of the Nine Energizing Breaths. Some are absolutely essential (the admonition against pregnant women practicing the exercises). Others are simply additional useful tips (time of day to practice, postural recommendations). And still others can be worked into your routine as your personal schedule permits (the number of saltwater baths you take each week).

1. Edwin Dingle recommended that the exercises be performed outside in the nude. This may work if you live in a remote area, but it is fine to perform them with loose, unrestricting clothing indoors. Do the routine with the windows open, if you can. Outside air is going to be fresher than indoor air.

2. Don't eat or drink anything cold for about an hour after performing the Nine Energizing Breaths. The exercises generate hot energy, and introducing cold into your body could cause a shock to the system. If you do it once or twice, it won't have a serious negative effect, but if you have, for instance, a glass of iced tea every morning after doing the Nine Energizing Breaths, within a couple of weeks, your energy system will become unbalanced, and your body will start feeling tired and worn out. It may also suppress your immune system and leave you more vulnerable to getting sick.

3. Since the Nine Energizing Breaths stimulate all the lower chakras, and especially the basic and sex chakras, it might be a bit too strong for teens to practice. It could overstimulate their sex drive.

4. Water will wash away prana, so if possible take your shower or bath before practicing, not after. To avoid washing away the full charge of the exercises, wait at least an hour or even two after practicing the routine before taking a shower or bath.

5. If meditation is part of your daily routine, you may want to perform the Nine Energizing Breaths following meditation. That's the optimal time to practice them. As you read earlier, the Nine Energizing Breaths strongly physicalize spiritual energy, which means that they actually infuse this high-quality prana into the body.

6. Try to take a saltwater bath at least twice a week in order to keep your energy body clean.

7. For additional Energetic Hygiene, make whatever modifications to your diet that you feel comfortable with. Reducing your consumption of meat would certainly help. Higher-level students of Arhatic Yoga typically adhere to a vegetarian diet, and Edwin Dingle himself advocated a regular "cleansing" diet that consisted of great quantities of fresh water and raw vegetables and fruits. The principle upon which these dietary recommendations is based is simple: the cleaner your food, the cleaner and higher-quality your energy.

8. Start out practicing in the morning until you see how much energy these exercises produce for you. If you perform them at night or even late in the afternoon, they may affect your sleep. But everyone reacts differently, so experiment with the time that works best for you.

9. If the Nine Energizing Breaths make you uncomfortable in any way, stop the routine and speak to your physician. Women who are pregnant or who think they may be pregnant should not perform the Nine Energizing Breaths. There's too much energy being generated for the unborn child.

10. If at any time during your practice, you feel edgy or you feel like your body is being overwhelmed with too much energy, stop your practice for a day or two. You may find it helpful to take more frequent saltwater baths.

11. Keep your spine straight throughout, during both the sitting and standing exercises. Your weight should be evenly distributed. You should be balanced and stable, but don't strain. Be aware of each muscle group in your body as you perform the exercises.

12. Do these exercises mindfully—that is, pay attention to your breathing and your body; don't perform them automatically. This isn't simply focused concentration; rather, it is placing light awareness on your actions. Focusing intently with your willpower actually inhibits your practice, as it will make you tense. Remember, the chi follows the yi; the energy will go where you intend it to go. And of course, with Nine

Energizing Breaths, you want your energy to be spread throughout your body. Thus, your intent, or awareness, for all the exercises should be on two things: first, the idea that you are now performing a set of exercises that will generate a tremendous amount of prana that will clean and energize your entire aura; and second, the specific area(s) that each exercise will clean and energize (see table 6.1 on page 93).

Reacquainting Myself with the Nine Energizing Breaths

I had chronic fatigue syndrome almost my entire life into early adulthood. During my surgical residency I recall working several thirty-two-hour on-call shifts a week and being absolutely depleted and exhausted by 10:00 a.m. on the morning of the first day (and then having to work through most of the night into the late afternoon on the following day taking care of very ill and demanding surgical trauma patients).

My life changed dramatically when I first met Master Co and told him about my condition, and he taught me the energy-generation exercises called the Five Tibetans, a short but powerful yoga routine also called the Five Tibetan Rites and the Tibetan Rejuvenation Rite. They gave me the jolt I really needed.

However, as the years went by, I found myself overworked and being pulled in too many directions. Family obligations and a busy urology and surgery practice were the main reasons. But, after my success with alternative healing methods became more widespread, I also found myself deluged with referrals from other physicians who sent me their most difficult cases—the ones that had resisted traditional medical treatment.

Suffice it to say, I had many demands on my time—and personal energy.

Throughout this period, I had relied on Grandmaster Choa's various meditations and energy-generation routines to help me keep up this pace. I had learned the Nine Energizing Breaths, but I tended to do the Five Tibetans more frequently, perhaps because I had learned them first.

I began to notice, though, that while the Five Tibetans would help jump-start me, I was getting more energetically congested—until it actually became quite an acute problem. I felt I needed a more evolved technique that would not only increase the energy levels in my body, but also clean out my energy channels and cause the prana to circulate and flow. So I meditated for guidance.

Shortly thereafter, as we focused on writing this book, I realized that I had drifted away from regular practice of the Nine Energizing Breaths. So I started them again, and by my second day of doing them, it seemed that they were the answer to my prayers. I felt the energy surge physically throughout my body, and yet at the same time, the energy channels in my body and particularly in my back felt open and flowing. The blockages (likely caused by an accumulation of emotional/stress energy) were gone. The increased amounts of energy were flowing freely. The first night that I did them, I was up half the night buzzing with a calm energy. The second day was pure bliss.

I truly believe that people will find the Nine Energizing Breaths to be an amazing gift.

ERIC B. ROBINS, MD

Exercise 6.1 **The Nine Energizing Breaths**
The First Energizing Breath

You may find this exercise going by several other names in other breathing or yoga systems, including Balancing Breathing, and in some Hindu teachings, Alternate Nasal Breathing. Perhaps most interesting, it is also sometimes referred to, in many yogic contexts, as Caduceus Breathing because of the way it helps to clean and energize the two energy channels, the ida and the pingala, that coil around the central energy channel of the torso, the sushumna, the way the two serpents coil around the staff of the caduceus symbol. The ida is connected to the left nostril and is associated with yin, or cooler energy, while the pingala is connected to the right nostril and is associated with yang, or warmer, energy. Also, the sushumna of Hindu or yogic systems corresponds to the "thrusting channel" in Chinese or Taoist teachings.

Thus, when you perform the First Energizing Breath, you are cleaning and synchronizing the flow of energy through these three key channels.

To Begin: You can either stand or sit for this exercise (most of the time in class, we have students stand, space permitting). Keep your feet flat on the floor and your spine straight. With your left hand relaxed, place your left thumb lightly against your left nostril. Place your tongue on your palate before you begin, and keep it there throughout the exercise.

Intent for the First Energizing Breath: Lightly put your awareness on the areas that you are going to clean and energize: the head and the brain. Remind yourself that you are going to balance the energy on both sides of the body.

Figure 6.1 **First Energizing Breath**

The First Energizing Breath: Exhale gently, through the mouth or the nose, until your lungs are empty. Close your left nostril with your left thumb, and perform a 6-count inhale through your right nostril. (One second per count is fine.) Close your right nostril with your left forefinger, and hold your breath for 3 counts. Remove your left thumb from your left nostril and exhale for 6 counts through the left nostril. Keeping your right nostril closed with your left forefinger, close your left nostril with your left thumb, and hold your exhale for 3 counts. Keeping your right nostril pinched shut, lift your thumb off your left nostril, and inhale for 6 counts through your left nostril. Then close your left nostril with your left thumb, and hold for 3 counts. Take your left forefinger off your right nostril and exhale for 6 counts. Close the right nostril again with your left forefinger, and hold your exhale for 3 counts. This sequence is one repetition. Repeat six more times for a total of seven cycles. Then just relax and take two normal breaths. See figure 6.1 for the entire sequence of movements for the First Energizing Breath.

Grandmaster Choa's modification for the First Energizing Breath: A more powerful rhythm and retention sequence. Edwin Dingle originally taught that students should inhale for 4 counts, hold for 16, exhale for 8, hold for 16, and so on. The 6-3-6-3-6-3 sequence is not only easier to remember and perform, it produces more prana.

Opening Clogged Nostrils and Relieving Sinus Congestion

If you experience occasional sinus congestion—as some people do in the morning—here's a solution: before you begin the First Energizing Breath, place a rolled-up towel or magazine firmly into the armpit opposite the clogged nostril. That is, if your left nostril is clogged, place the rolled-up towel under your right armpit. This will put pressure on the energy channel that controls your nasal passages; your congestion should be relieved shortly.

The Second Energizing Breath

The Second Energizing Breath, sometimes called Rapid Turtle Breathing in other systems, cleans your head and brain. It also gives you the ability to think clearly. When clairvoyants observe someone performing this breath, they see the brain getting whiter and brighter, almost luminous.

To perform the Second Energizing Breath, you can either stand or sit. In class, we have students stand, space permitting, because you get more complete cleaning action when you stand. If you sit, the exercise cleans down to your waist or basic chakra. However, when you stand, you can clean and energize down your entire back and to your heels.

To Begin: Keep your feet flat on the floor and your spine straight. With shoulders relaxed, let your head droop until your chin rests on your chest. Place your tongue on your palate as you begin, but for this exercise and this exercise only, there is a time during which you will be instructed to remove it from your palate.

Intent for the Second Energizing Breath: Lightly put your awareness on the areas that you are going to clean and energize: the head, neck, spine, and back.

The Second Energizing Breath: Note that both your inhale and exhale in this exercise should be quicker and more vigorous than in the First Energizing Breath. Begin by exhaling, through your mouth or nose, until your lungs are empty. Then inhale through both nostrils, and as you do so, raise your head off your chest, pivoting backward at the neck. Move your head up and back as far as it can comfortably go. Don't strain. Coordinate your inhalation so that when your lungs are full, your head is all the way back.

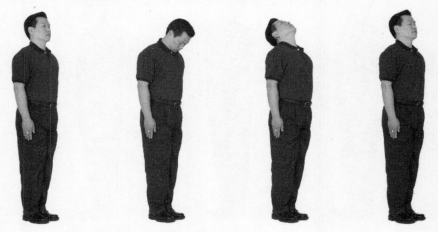

Figure 6.2 **Second Energizing Breath**

After your head is all the way back, pause for a moment; then exhale through the mouth, and as you do, swing your head forward, gently pivoting at the neck, back to the starting position. Remove your tongue from your palate as you exhale. This is done to create an easier and more natural movement and to enable you to exhale more forcefully, which gets rid of more dirty energy. This is the only time in your practice of the Nine Energizing Breaths that you will take your tongue off the palate. Your exhale should be forceful and audible, but your face and cheeks should not be tense. As you exhale, your cheeks should puff out a bit, and you should hear your breath ("ssshhh"). Time your exhale so that, as your lungs become empty, your chin has returned to the starting position on your chest. Breathe vigorously, but don't overdo it. You don't want to hyperventilate. This is one repetition. Repeat thirteen more times so that you do a set of 14 breaths total. Pause and take 2 normal breaths. Then do a second set of 14 breaths, pause again, and take 2 normal breaths. Perform a third set of 14 breaths followed by a pause and 2 normal breaths. Close by performing a fourth set of just 7 breaths. When you are finished, simply relax and take 2 normal breaths. See figure 6.2 for the entire sequence of movements for the Second Energizing Breath.

Grandmaster Choa's modification for the Second Energizing Breath: A different number of repetitions and sets, while keeping the total number of breaths the same. Edwin Dingle instructed students to perform seven sets of 7, but 14-14-14-7 generates more prana.

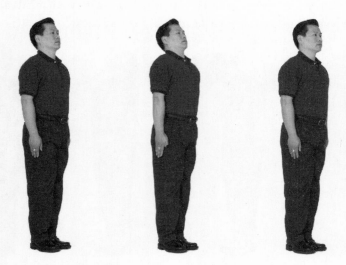

Figure 6.3 **Third Energizing Breath**

The Third Energizing Breath

The Third Energizing Breath cleans, energizes, and activates the chakras of the entire body. While the first two breaths focus on cleaning the head, spine, and several major channels of the energetic anatomy, this breath begins to push the energy through the rest of the meridians and out into the extremities.

To Begin: Perform this exercise standing. Be firm but not tense. Keep your head straight, your face forward, and your back straight. Keep your feet straight with your heels together. Keep your arms and hands at your sides with your elbows lightly locked. Keep your fingers together and your mouth closed. Place your tongue on your palate before you begin, and keep it there throughout the exercise.

Intent for the Third Energizing Breath: Remind yourself that you are going to forcefully energize the entire body. Lightly put your awareness on driving the energy up from the lower part of the body and out into the arms and legs.

The Third Energizing Breath: Begin by exhaling gently through your mouth until your lungs are comfortably empty. Then begin a deep inhalation through your nose. Fill your lungs completely. After your lungs are full, take a final vigorous and audible inhalation through the nose, and then "lock in" the breath by tensing all the muscles of your body: neck, jaw, back, arms, legs, torso, and buttocks. Feel your muscles flex and your body get rigid. Don't strain, though; the veins on your neck and temples should not be bulging. The last muscle group you should squeeze is your pubococcygeal or PC muscles. This is the set of muscles that runs from the front of the pubic bone back to the anus and controls your urinary and bowel movement functions. When you squeeze this chain of muscles, it is the same contraction you would use to prevent yourself from going to the bathroom both front and back. While holding your breath, keep your body tense for five seconds. Exhale, relax your body, and take 2 normal breaths. Repeat. See figure 6.3 for the entire sequence of movements for the Third Energizing Breath.

Grandmaster Choa's modification for the Third through Ninth Energizing Breaths: It's the PC squeeze. Edwin Dingle's original full routine would take about an hour to complete. But Grandmaster Choa's addition of squeezing the PC muscles during the Third through the Ninth Energizing Breaths generates and drives so much prana throughout the entire body that the whole routine can be completed in about ten minutes.

The Fourth Energizing Breath

The Fourth Energizing Breath follows up on the focus of the Third, in that it continues to push the energy throughout the large and small meridians of the body. However, it also has a particular focus on the chakras of the upper body, especially the front and back heart chakras.

To Begin: Use the same position as for the Third Energizing Breath.

Intent for the Fourth Energizing Breath: Lightly put your awareness on the areas that you are going to clean and energize: the upper part of the torso, and especially the front and back heart chakras.

The Fourth Energizing Breath: Exhale gently through the mouth until your lungs are empty. As you inhale through the nose, swing your arms smoothly in an arc out to your sides and overhead. Keep your elbows and wrists lightly locked as you raise your arms. Your palms remain down throughout. Coordinate your movement with your breathing so that when your lungs are full, your arms are directly overhead, and the backs

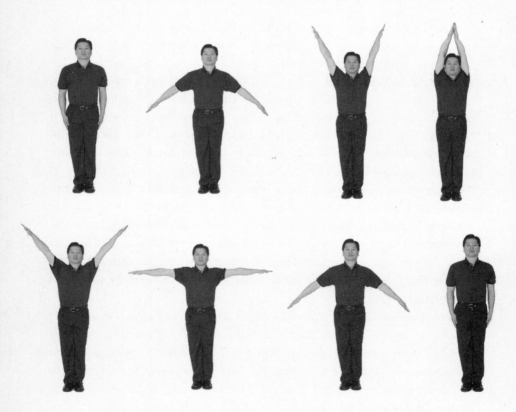

Figure 6.4 **Fourth Energizing Breath**

of your hands are touching. After your lungs are full, as you did with the Third Energizing Breath, take one final vigorous inhalation through the nose, and then lock in the breath by tensing all the muscles of your body, especially the PC muscles. Hold your breath and this tensed posture for five seconds. Then release your breath in three short, sharp exhalations through clenched teeth as you bring your arms down along the same arc you used to raise them: arms at 2:00 and 10:00 (first exhalation); arms at 3:00 and 9:00 (second exhalation); arms at 4:00 and 8:00 (third exhalation). As your hands return to your thighs, release any remaining breath; then relax your body and take 2 normal breaths. Repeat. See figure 6.4 for the entire sequence of movements for the Fourth Energizing Breath.

The Fifth Energizing Breath

The Fifth Energizing Breath is a very smooth movement that focuses on the chakras of the upper body, particularly the throat chakra, the front and back heart chakras, and the front and back spleen chakras. Physically, it loosens up the muscles of the neck, shoulders, and upper back. Many practitioners report feeling a melting sensation during this breath. This is the chakras being charged.

To Begin: Use the same position as for the Third Energizing Breath.

Intent for the Fifth Energizing Breath: Lightly put your awareness on the areas that you are going to clean and energize: the upper half of the body and the upper chakras, from the solar plexus up to the crown.

The Fifth Energizing Breath: Exhale through the mouth until your lungs are empty. As you inhale through the nose, make two vertical fists (thumbs on top), and raise your arms to shoulder height directly in front of you. Keep your wrists and elbows lightly locked. After your lungs are full, take one final vigorous inhalation through the nose, and then lock in the

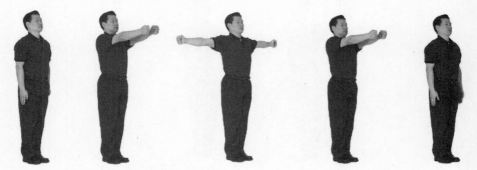

Figure 6.5 **Fifth Energizing Breath**

breath by tensing all the muscles of your body, including the PC muscles. While holding your breath and keeping your body tense, swing your arms out to the side parallel to the ground until your body forms a T. Then, swing your arms back to shoulder height in front of you. Perform this butterfly motion two more times (three times total). Then bring your hands down to your sides, relax your fists, and exhale. Relax and take 2 normal breaths. Repeat. See figure 6.5 for the entire sequence of movements for the Fifth Energizing Breath.

The Sixth Energizing Breath

The Sixth and Seventh Energizing Breaths have large, powerful, dynamic movements that really stir up and expel the dirty energy of the aura. As you perform them, don't get carried away to the point of losing correct form, but don't be afraid to really get into them. These aren't delicate movements. Physically, this exercise loosens up the muscles of the shoulders, neck, and upper body.

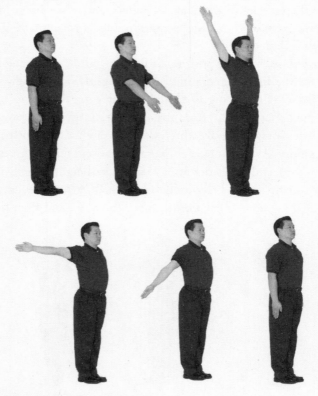

Figure 6.6 **Sixth Energizing Breath**

To Begin: Use the same position as for the Third Energizing Breath.

Intent for the Sixth Energizing Breath: Similar to the Fifth Energizing Breath. Lightly put your awareness on the areas that you are going to clean and energize: the entire body, and especially the front and back solar plexus chakras.

The Sixth Energizing Breath: Exhale through the mouth until your lungs are empty. Then, as you have already learned to do in the previous exercises, inhale fully, tense your body, lock in your breath, and lock the PC muscle group. As you hold your breath and muscular tension, pivot your arms outward and upward. Continue with that movement, swinging your arms smoothly in an arc that will take them over your head and behind you. Keep the wrists, elbows, and shoulders firm throughout. Your goal is to move your arms backward roughly in a circle, and then to return them to the starting position. Unless you're really flexible, you won't be able to make a full circle, but that's okay. The movement should not be uncomfortable or painful. While continuing to hold your breath and keep your body tense, do two more circular motions for a total of three repetitions. Then return to your starting position. Relax your body and take 2 normal breaths. Repeat. See figure 6.6 for the entire sequence of movements for the Sixth Energizing Breath.

The Seventh Energizing Breath

The Seventh Energizing Breath, like the Sixth, is a dynamic, sweeping movement. The difference with the Seventh is that your hands begin and end at the small of the back (meng mein chakra). Thus, it helps accumulate and clean away stress energy from the lower back; that's the purpose of the little wiping motion at the end of the exercise.

To Begin: Use the same position as for the Third Energizing Breath. Then place your hands behind you at the meng mein (roughly the belt line), palms facing backward with your thumbs and forefingers touching. Your hands will form an open diamond shape at the belt line. See the first and sixth pictures in figure 6.7 for details. Bend your elbows, but still keep the arms slightly tense. Your shoulders will be forced back slightly and your chest out.

Intent for the Seventh Energizing Breath: Lightly put your awareness on the areas that you are going to clean and energize: the upper chakras—from the solar plexus up to the crown—and the head, neck, shoulders, and arms.

The Seventh Energizing Breath: Exhale through the mouth until your lungs are empty. Inhale fully; then lock in your breath, lock the PC muscle

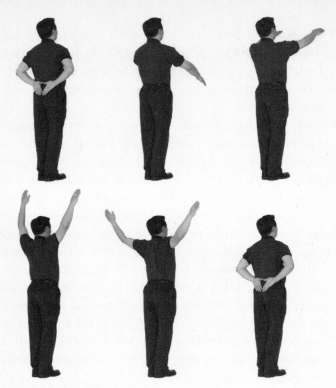

Figure 6.7 **Seventh Energizing Breath**

group, and tense your body, as you have already learned to do in the previous exercises. Hold your breath and tension as you unlock your hands and swing your arms forward, raising them overhead in the same way you did in the Sixth Energizing Breath. Keep your wrists and elbows slightly tense throughout the movement. As you bring your hands back to the original position, reposition the left hand into the right. Perform two more circular movements for a total of three. After the third repetition, flick your hands downward, wiping away dirty energy from the lower back. Then exhale, relax, and take 2 normal breaths. Repeat. See figure 6.7 for the entire sequence of movements for the Seventh Energizing Breath.

The Eighth Energizing Breath

The Eighth Energizing Breath has a strong cleansing and energizing effect on the entire aura and physical body, as it exercises two key pumping stations for prana moving from the lower chakras to the upper chakras: the meng mein chakra and the back of the neck. The movement of the head up and down and bending from the waist help to open these important areas of the spine.

To Begin: Use the same position as for the Third Energizing Breath. Then place your hands on the crest of your hip bones so that your thumbs reach for your kidneys and your fingers spread across your abdomen. If you can move your elbows forward slightly without discomfort, do so. If any part of this beginning posture is uncomfortable, though, just do the exercise with your hands on your hips.

Intent for the Eighth Energizing Breath: Lightly put your awareness on the areas that you are going to clean and energize: the trunk, head, and brain; also the lower abdomen, sex chakra, and throat chakra.

The Eighth Energizing Breath: Exhale through the mouth until your lungs are empty. Inhale completely, lock in your breath, lock the PC muscle group, and tense your body, as you have already learned to do in the previous exercises. As you hold your breath and bodily tension, roll your head gently forward as far as it can comfortably go; then move it back as far as it will comfortably go. While still holding your breath, do this movement two more times. After your third repetition, bring your

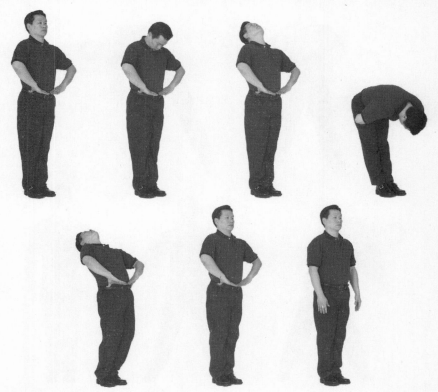

Figure 6.8 **Eighth Energizing Breath**

head back to the starting position and exhale fully. Then, without inhaling and while maintaining your bodily tension, bend forward from the hips as far as you can comfortably go, trying to get your upper body parallel to the floor; then bend backward as far as you can comfortably go. Do this movement two more times, for a total of three times. Then, return to the starting posture. Relax and take 2 normal breaths. Repeat. See figure 6.8 for the entire sequence of movements for the Eighth Energizing Breath.

The Ninth Energizing Breath

The Ninth Energizing Breath ties together all the previous exercises by cleaning and balancing the entire aura and all the chakras. It also emphasizes "rooting power," or using the chakras of the soles of the feet to connect to the energy of the earth.

To Begin: Use the same position as the Eighth Energizing Breath, except keep your feet shoulder-width apart.

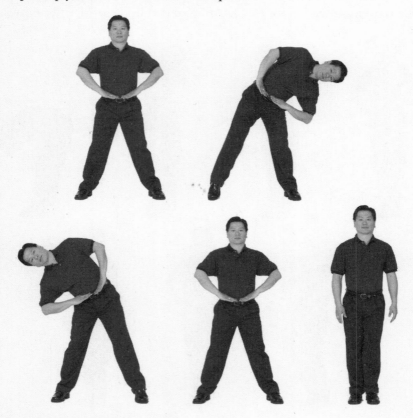

Figure 6.9 **Ninth Energizing Breath**

Intent for the Ninth Energizing Breath: Remind yourself that you are going to clean, energize, and balance your entire body and aura. Lightly put your awareness on your entire body.

The Ninth Energizing Breath: Exhale through the mouth until your lungs are empty. Inhale fully, then lock in your breath, lock the PC muscle group, and tense your body, as you have already learned to do in the previous exercises. As you hold your breath and bodily tension, pivot sideways from the hip, leaning over to the left as far as you comfortably can, until your right heel slightly comes off the ground. Then perform the movement in the other direction, bending to the left, until your right heel comes slightly off the ground. Do this two more times, for a total of three times to each side. Then bring your hands back to the sides of your body, exhale, and relax. Take 2 normal breaths. Repeat. See figure 6.9 for the entire sequence of movements for the Ninth Energizing Breath.

* * *

After you complete the Nine Energizing Breaths, you are ready to meet the day, fully charged up. Simply walk around and stretch a bit. Just remember the admonition about not eating or drinking anything cold right afterward. Also, remember Grandmaster Choa's principle of moderation. It's not unusual for people to feel so "buzzed"—particularly if they're used to feeling run-down—that they begin to question if what they're feeling is actually real: "Am I really feeling energized? Am I imagining this? Is it going to run out soon?" If you find yourself getting excited about your newfound energy, try to simply relax and enjoy it. One good suggestion is to do something constructive with it. Attack a personal project that's been lingering or that you've been dragging your feet about. Do something nice for someone else. Be of service. (Pranic healers often use the Nine Energizing Breaths just before a healing session to charge themselves up, or just after the session to recharge.)

Finally, simply realize that you did it yourself; you just found a simple, easy way to give yourself a jolt. You can use the energy for whatever positive purpose you want. And perhaps best of all, you can do the Nine Energizing Breaths again tomorrow morning and feel the same way!

Pranic Healing, Arhatic Yoga, and Mentalphysics

We wrote earlier of the root teachings connection between Mentalphysics and Pranic Healing and Arhatic Yoga. There are many ways in which the two systems complement each other. In ancient times, to prevent misuse of powerful information, those who possessed great spiritual wisdom—whether they were monks affiliated with temples, yogis moving from town to town, hermits living apart from a village, or simply wise men moving among the people—were reluctant to impart to any one school or disciple the entire canon of esoteric knowledge. As a result, many schools would have a "part" of the whole, and their part would be passed down to the students. It would be up to enterprising students to seek out knowledge to fill in the gaps, a quest that might take a lifetime or even many lifetimes.

Pranic Healing is an ancient system of energy healing modified for the modern world. Arhatic Yoga is a distillation of powerfully effective ancient yogic meditations. The Nine Energizing Breaths, derived from the original Mentalphysics breathing exercises, are a powerful energy-generation program with equally deep ancient esoteric roots.

Thus, when someone practices Pranic Healing, Arhatic Yoga, and the Nine Energizing Breaths, he or she is filling in one of those ancient gaps. Together, they comprise a complete system of spiritual practices, meditation, and energy-generation and healing for mind, body, and spirit.

Part Four

Advanced Practices

for Enhanced Purification

and Sustained Energy

Chapter 7 Meditation

Jen Bowlin of St. Louis suffers from several medical ailments, including narcolepsy, asthma, Ehlers-Danlos syndrome, migraines, rosacea, GERD, and arthritis. On top of that, she was hospitalized after an adverse reaction to a medication. Nonetheless, she learned and began to practice the Nine Energizing Breaths every morning, even though, as she notes, "When I began, I couldn't raise my arms above my head without pain, dizziness, and shortness of breath. Gradually my condition improved and after three months I was able to decrease my medications and my vision improved. I continue to do the exercises and grow spiritually. I am thankful to have learned them".

Our English word "meditation" is derived from the Latin verb *meditari*, which means "to think over, to consider, or to ponder." In general usage, it refers to deep, often solitary, reflection on a topic; to meditate on something is to give it serious thought. However, throughout the history of Western thought and particularly Christian theology, the word also became associated with prayer and contemplation. And over the last fifty years, with the growing acceptance of Eastern thought, we have begun to understand meditation as a mental exercise that helps us let go of our conscious thoughts and calm the mind. Thus, meditation today has a multitude of meanings in a variety of contexts.

For our purposes in this book, though, we will look to the definition offered by Grandmaster Choa Kok Sui, which is more in line with meditation as traditionally conceived in Eastern philosophy. Meditation is "either prolonged awareness or spiritual practice."[1] The Sanskrit word for such an exercise is *sadhana*, which refers literally to spiritual practices undertaken with an eye toward a specific goal—in most cases, enlightenment or oneness.

To understand this true sense of meditation clearly, you need to understand the difference between several terms that are often confused. The first is *concentration,* which is a function of willpower. Concentration is "prolonged focusing" or "prolonged one-pointedness." It's the ability to keep your mind or attention on one thing for a period of time. This is different from passively staring at a TV screen and being so absorbed by the program you're watching that you don't hear someone calling your name. Concentration is willful direction of your attention. The second term is *awareness,* for which we in the Western world, at least with regard to meditation, have no true corresponding word. In most Western connotations, *awareness* is used as a synonym for understanding or knowing (for example, "He's aware that it's going to rain tomorrow") or to describe a state of vigilance or alertness to your external surroundings or circumstances (for example, "A pilot has to maintain awareness of a multitude of factors when coming in for a landing"). Neither definition really gets to the notion of awareness as it relates to meditation, which in Sanskrit is more properly the term *dhyana,* which means "prolonged sensitivity."

In Grandmaster Choa's conception, meditation also includes a third element, *stillness,* which refers to calming the mind and, especially, any negative emotions, such as fears or anxieties, that may be stirring around in there. Stillness is better understood by practicing it than reading a description of it, but it is achieved by turning off the thoughts and noting the lack of sensory impressions in your mind, sensing an "inner void"; it's letting go.

Thus, meditation, as discussed here, is a type of spiritual practice (a sadhana) that both includes and balances prolonged one-pointedness and prolonged awareness, and also creates inner stillness.

The meditations that we include here all incorporate the notions of one-pointedness, awareness, and stillness, but at a fairly basic level, for these are meditations designed to be performed without personal instruction and guidance. (It is always advisable to practice advanced meditations only under the direction of a competent teacher.) However, while they are simple to learn and perform, they are still effective and powerful. And when combined with the Nine Energizing Breaths, they have an even more potent cleansing and energizing effect on your mind and body.

Also, these are all yin meditations; they don't generate hard, strong energy the way many of the yang meditations of Arhatic Yoga do. These produce more loving, receptive energy; they clean your aura and open your heart and crown chakras. This makes them ideal for general meditation purposes and also an effective complement to the very yang Nine Energizing Breaths.

The meditations included here are Meditation on Twin Hearts, which is the truly special foundational meditation of Grandmaster Choa Kok Sui's system; the Dissolving into Light Meditation, which works on both the physical and energetic levels to heal the body and increase your connection with the Higher Soul; and the Revitalizing Meditation, which recharges and revitalizes all the chakras and meridians of your energy body, as well as the organs, glands, and structure of your physical body.

GENERAL MEDITATION TIPS

Here are some general tips that apply to all the meditations in this chapter. It's best to meditate on an empty stomach. Then wait at least thirty minutes after meditating before eating. This allows your body to focus on assimilating the prana rather than eating and digesting food. Also, don't drink anything cold for one hour before and one hour after meditating. The energy that you generate is warm, and cold drinks may either negate the energy you've produced or unnecessarily jolt your energy channels. As you read in chapter 6, "Performing the Nine Energizing Breaths," introducing cold substances into a body that has generated warm meditation or the Nine Energizing Breaths energy can shock the system. Don't meditate in direct sunlight because the solar prana is too strong. Don't meditate when you're feeling angry or fearful or when you're experiencing any strong negative emotion. Don't take a shower for at least ninety minutes after meditating. As you read earlier, water washes away prana. Don't resist outside distractions, such as noises, and even more important, don't get angry at them. If you hear a dog barking or a phone ringing, don't react. Simply acknowledge the distraction, and then bring your mind back to whatever point you are at in your meditation.

MEDITATION FORMAT: STEPS COMMON TO ALL THE MEDITATIONS

There is a certain format to these meditations that you will follow, particularly at the beginning and ending of each. So the meditation format will look like this: certain common steps at the beginning, then the meditation proper, then certain common steps at the end.

At the beginning:

1. Begin with Cleansing Physical Exercises (see chapter 5). Perform at least one set (and preferably two sets) of the Cleansing Physical

Exercises before meditating to prepare the energy body to receive additional prana.

2. Sit quietly and comfortably in a chair that gives your body support, but don't rest against the back of the chair. Leaning back tends to cause your posture to slump as the meditation proceeds, and this partially compresses the spine, which obstructs the flow of energy.

3. Rest your hands in your lap, palms up. While some meditations call for various *mudras*, or hand postures with certain fingers touching—and other, more advanced Arhatic Yoga meditations do employ mudras—for these basic meditations, simply keep your hands apart and palms up, resting in your lap. Palms up is a general hand posture for receiving energy, and it is suitable for any meditation.

4. Place your tongue on your palate, as you read in chapter 3 when you learned about pranic breathing, and keep it there throughout the meditation. This connects the two large energy channels of your body and greatly facilitates the smooth flow of prana throughout the body.

5. Invoke. We always invoke, or offer a brief prayer, at the beginning of a meditation for divine guidance, blessing, and protection. Everyone has a different spiritual orientation, so feel free to use the invocations offered here or one of your own choosing. But you should definitely invoke at the outset of meditation.

Specific meditation: After these five beginning steps, you will perform the meditation proper.

At the end:

1. Perform blessing and rooting or grounding. Meditation builds up a lot of energy in your aura and physical body. In order to avoid energetic congestion—and also to use the energy accumulated for a positive purpose—we bless our loved ones, life circumstances (for example, job or career, special projects), and the earth at the conclusion of each meditation. Blessing the earth, also called *rooting* or *grounding,* not only enables us to bless the earth but also to strengthen our energetic attachment to it. Rooting involves simply visualizing prana radiating

downward from the soles of your feet and the base of the spine ten feet or more into the earth. This increases your attachment to the earth—literally grounding you—and helps you avoid the spacey feeling that sometimes follows deep or intense meditations.

2. Give thanks. This is simply a closing prayer, using a shortened version of the invocation language.

3. Stand up and perform one set of the Nine Energizing Breaths. This will prevent energetic congestion and also help assimilate the fresh prana generated during meditation that's floating around in your aura into your physical body. You can also perform other physical routines after meditation, including the Cleansing Physical Exercises, but it would be good for your practice to get into the habit of performing the Nine Energizing Breaths regularly.

MEDITATION ON TWIN HEARTS

Grandmaster Choa Kok Sui's Meditation on Twin Hearts[2] is an amazing and unique meditation. Working on every level of the mind, body, and spirit, this brief (twenty-minute) meditation opens first the heart chakra (the physical heart), then the crown chakra (the spiritual heart), and finally both simultaneously. The result is an aura purged of negative emotions and injurious thoughts, and a mind cleared of distractions and filled with peace.

Practiced regularly before performing the Nine Energizing Breaths, this meditation flushes dirty energy from the aura and replaces it with fresh, clean prana. When you perform Meditation on Twin Hearts, a clairvoyant sees a great flood of white light pouring into the crown, erasing the dark smudges of negative thought forms in your aura, and then flowing out to fill and illuminate the entire energy body. After the aura is cleansed, its overall level of prana is balanced and can flow unimpeded, which can promote physical healing. It can also lead to a better, more positive outlook because when your aura is filled with negative thought forms, it's like looking at the world through a dirty windshield. Remember, you're inside your aura, so it's the lens through which you see the world.

When the crown is opened and the downflow of energy rushes in through it, many people also experience what is called "inner illumination." This manifests differently for everyone, but most describe it as a feeling of deep inner stillness and peace. The second part of Meditation on Twin Hearts helps bring about this illumination by directing you to meditate on the "OM" sound (a universal mantra, or sound, of divine peace), and the gap or the space between the OMs for several minutes. Meditating on this gap is the key, as it produces a state of inner stillness during which many people are able to make contact with their Higher Soul.

OM is probably the most well-known mantra used by meditators today. Also written *aum,* it is a universal sound that is Hindu in origin but has correlations in many other cultures as well. For instance, the Christian *amen* is a version of OM, as is the Muslim *amin.* Regardless of the spiritual tradition, the sound has a powerful purifying effect on the aura during meditation and helps the meditator elevate his or her consciousness to a higher level, partly because the sound is a meditation on some of the attributes of God: *Om*niscient, *Om*nipresent, *Om*nipotent, and so on. The sound can also be used to purify or cleanse objects or rooms. For instance, you can play an OM CD repeatedly in a room to dispel dirty energy. In addition to its usage here in Meditation on Twin Hearts, OM is used prominently in several Arhatic Yoga meditations, including Achieving Oneness with the Higher Soul, and OM Mani Padme Hum.

On a different level, Meditation on Twin Hearts enables those who are so inclined to render service—by becoming better healers of others and helping to heal the planet. In opening first the heart chakra and then the crown chakra via this meditation, a person begins to develop a greater sense of compassion for all beings on the planet. As that compassion grows, the person develops similarly positive character traits: mercy, understanding, acceptance, and forgiveness. The growth of these positive emotions further opens the crown chakra and even more divine spiritual energy can flow in. The size and diameter of the spiritual cord, the thread that connects the Higher Soul to the Incarnated Soul (in the body), continues to increase, and the person's spiritual development is further accelerated. As a result of these energetic and emotional changes, the person will begin to have more high-quality prana available for healing others when employing Pranic Healing, and for healing the planet when practicing Meditation on Twin Hearts.

Additionally, the development of positive character traits such as compassion, mercy, and forgiveness helps to "immunize" the aura against energetic contamination from the negativity of others. It's an energetic rule that "like attracts like," and as you begin to minimize—and hopefully, eliminate—negative emotions such as anger and resentment through regular practice of Meditation on Twin Hearts, the anger of others will have nothing to "grab on to" in your aura. When someone tries to provoke you or "push your buttons," outwardly, you'll just appear more calm; you simply won't react or get angry. Inwardly, energetically, there is no negative energy in your aura for the projected negative emotions of others to mix with and react to. Meditation on Twin Hearts can have a profound effect on those practicing it. "Meditation on Twin Hearts is fantastic for experiencing inner stillness," says Shana Hildebrand of Los Angeles. "Since I have been practicing on a regular basis, I have found not only has my emotional state in general become more peaceful, but I also have this wonderful internal calmness. It is a priceless gift."

Exercise 7.1 **Meditation on Twin Hearts**

There are two ways you can do this meditation: you can either follow the numbered steps below, or you can listen to a Meditation on Twin Hearts CD prepared by Grandmaster Choa Kok Sui. It's the same meditation, but with the CD, you have the benefit of having Grandmaster Choa guide you through it. (See Contact Information on page 187 for how to obtain a Meditation on Twin Hearts CD.) If you follow the steps below, you may want to read the entire meditation through several times so that you understand the various steps.

Here are a few brief tips on performing this meditation. People with high blood pressure, heart problems, or glaucoma should not perform Meditation on Twin Hearts. The energy may aggravate those conditions. In particular, the front and back heart chakras and the meng mein chakra all become highly activated, and these chakras are associated with the circulatory system. Additionally, the meng mein regulates your blood pressure. Women who are pregnant or who think they may be pregnant should not perform Meditation on Twin Hearts. The energy may be unsafe for an unborn child. Those under the age of eighteen should not practice the illumination technique (the second part of the meditation), as the energy produced may be too much for their not-yet-mature bodies. During the blessing portion, perform the blessings with true emotion; don't just do them perfunctorily. Work on really feeling the feelings of love you call up when you bless the earth. See smiling faces. Visualize an earth of peace, love, and joy. See people living together in harmony. Visualizing a golden-pinkish light flowing from your hands to the earth is also helpful.

Let's begin the meditation.

1. **Cleanse the energy body through physical exercise.** Do the Cleansing Physical Exercises for five to ten minutes (one or two sets) to cleanse and prepare your aura.

2. **Sit quietly in a chair with your hands in your lap, palms up. Connect your tongue to your palate.**

3. **Invocation for divine blessing.** Close your eyes. You can make your own invocation. For instance, Hindus can pray to Shiva or Krishna or to the Guru; Christians to Jesus Christ, or Mary; Muslims to Allah; and Buddhists to Buddha. If you are eclectic, you may say, "To the Universal Supreme God." Here is one general invocation suitable for all:

> To the Supreme God,
> To my spiritual teacher, to all the spiritual teachers,
> To the holy angels and spiritual helpers,
> And all the Great Ones,
> We humbly invoke divine guidance,
> Divine love, illumination, divine oneness,
> Divine bliss, divine help, and divine protection.
> We thank you in full faith.

4. **Activate the heart chakra by blessing the entire earth with loving-kindness.** Press your front heart chakra with your finger for a few seconds to make concentration easier on the front heart chakra. Then, think about an image or feeling that generates for you the emotions of love and joy. Perhaps it's your spouse or child; perhaps it's another person or image very close to you. Use a visualization or picture that enables you to feel those feelings.

   Raise your hands at chest level with your palms facing outward. Visualize the earth as a small ball in front of you. Concentrate on and be aware of the front heart chakra, and feel those feelings of love and joy as you bless the earth with loving-kindness. Blessing the earth should not be done mechanically, but with feeling. You may use the prayer of St. Francis of Assisi (which is what Grandmaster Choa uses on his Meditation on Twin Hearts CD). Be aware of your heart as you silently say the following:

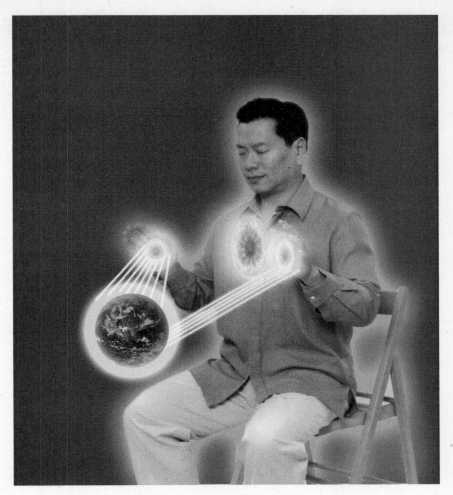

Figure 7.1 **Meditation on Twin Hearts, Blessing through the Heart**

Lord, make me an instrument of your peace.

Feel the inner peace within you. Allow yourself to be a channel of divine peace. Feel the peace within you. Let it flow to your arms, to your hands. You may visualize warm, pink light flowing from your heart through your arms and out through your palms to the small earth in front of you. Bless the earth with peace. Gently and lovingly share this peace.

Where there is hatred, let me sow love.

Feel the divine love within you. Allow yourself to be a channel of divine love. Feel this love within you. Feel this love flowing from your heart to your arms and to your hands, flowing to the small earth in front of you. Bless the earth with peace and with love (see figure 7.1).

Where there is injury, pardon.

Feel the spirit of reconciliation. Allow yourself to be a channel of divine forgiveness and divine reconciliation. Bless the earth with the spirit of forgiveness, reconciliation,understanding, harmony, and peace.

Where there is doubt, faith; where there is despair, hope.

Feel divine hope and faith. Allow yourself to be a channel of divine hope and faith. Bless the earth with hope and faith. In particular, you may want to bless parts of the world that have suffered or are suffering from war or natural disasters. Bless people who are having a difficult time with hope and faith. Silently tell those affected, "You can make it." Bless them with divine hope, divine faith, and divine strength.

Where there is darkness, light; where there is sadness, joy.

Allow yourself to be a channel of divine light and joy. Bless the entire earth with divine light and joy. Bless people who are sad, depressed, and in pain with light and joy. Fill them with light and joy.

When blessing, feel and appreciate the implications of each phrase. You may also use visualization. As you bless the earth with loving-kindness, visualize the aura of the earth becoming dazzling golden pink. This blessing can be directed to a nation or group of nations. Do not direct this blessing to specific infants, children, or other persons during the main meditation because they might be overwhelmed by the energy. You may bless them after releasing the excess energy.

5. **Activate the crown chakra by blessing the earth with loving-kindness.** Press the crown with your finger for several seconds to facilitate concentration on the crown chakra, and bless the entire earth with loving-kindness. You may visualize a warm golden light flowing from your crown down through your arms and out

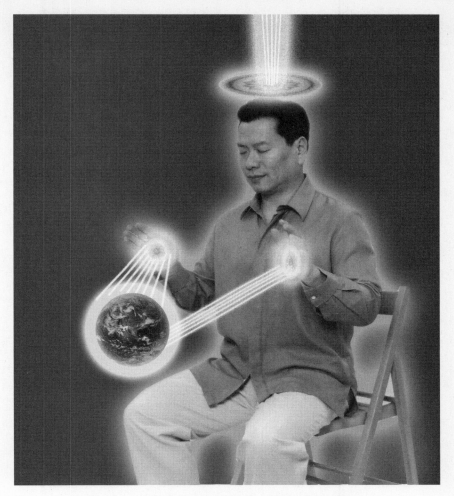

Figure 7.2 **Meditation on Twin Hearts, Blessing through the Crown**

your hands to the small earth in front of you (see figure 7.2). The
following blessing may be used:

> From the center of the heart of God,
>   Let the entire earth be blessed
>   With loving-kindness.

Feel the divine love and kindness. Allow yourself to be a channel of
divine love and kindness and share these with the whole earth.

Let the entire earth be blessed with
Great joy and happiness.

Feel the joy and happiness and share these with the entire earth. Visualize people smiling, their hearts filled with joy and happiness.

From the center of the heart of God,
Let the entire earth be blessed with
Understanding, harmony, and divine peace.

Allow yourself to be a channel of understanding, harmony, and peace. Visualize people or nations that are fighting (or are on the verge of fighting) reconciling and living in harmony with each other. Visualize people putting down their arms, shaking hands, and embracing each other.

Let the entire earth be blessed with
Goodwill and the will to do good.

Imagine people not only filled with good intentions and talking about doing something good but actually carrying out these good intentions and performing good deeds. This is the meaning of the "will to do good."

6. **Meditate and bless the earth with loving-kindness simultaneously through the heart and crown chakras.** Now, simultaneously concentrate on and be aware of both the crown and heart chakras, and bless the earth with loving-kindness through both chakras for a few minutes. This will align both chakras, thereby making the blessing much more potent. Visualize a golden light from your hands going down to the earth, filling the whole earth with light and love (see figure 7.3).
    You may use this blessing:

From the center of the heart of God,
Let the entire earth, every person, and every being
Be blessed with divine love and kindness.

Feel the divine love and kindness, and share these with the whole earth, every person, and every being.

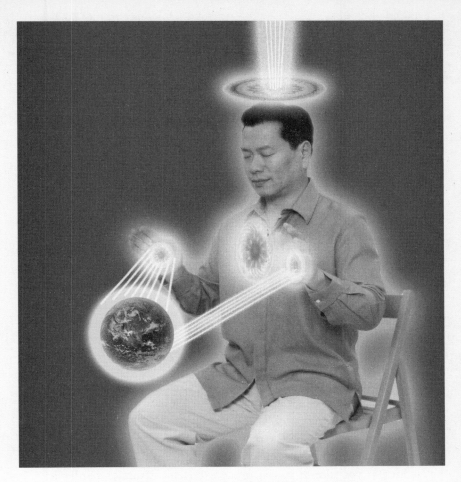

Figure 7.3 **Meditation on Twin Hearts, Blessing through the Heart and Crown Simultaneously**

Let the entire earth, every person,
And every being be blessed
With divine sweetness, divine joy
With warmness, caring, and tenderness.

Feel the sweet, loving feeling, and share it with the whole earth.

From the center of the heart of God,
Let the entire earth, every person, and every being
Be blessed with inner healing, inner beauty,
Divine bliss, and divine oneness.

Feel the divine bliss and divine oneness, and share these with every person and every being.

7. **The second part of the meditation is the illumination technique. Meditate on the light, on the mantra OM, and on the intervals between the OMs.** Put your hands down. Gently imagine a brilliant white light or golden light on the crown chakra. Look at it gently and lovingly. Feel the quality of the energy emitted by the light. Feel the inner peace, stillness, and bliss emanating from the light (see figure 7.4). Be aware of the light, the inner stillness, and the bliss. After you can clearly see this point of light, begin chanting to yourself silently the mantra OM. Pronounce it slowly, purposefully and silently:

> Oooommmm . . . oooommmm . . . oooommmm . . .
> Oooommmm . . . oooommmm . . . oooommmm . . .
> Oooommmm . . . oooommmm . . . oooommmm . . .

Breathe slowly. Throughout the illumination technique, keep your awareness on the point of light, the OM sound, and also the silence or gap between the OMs. You can continue like this for about five to ten minutes. Then, let your mind go blank. Stop the visualization of the light and the mantra, and just let go. For a few minutes simply let yourself feel the feeling of inner peace and stillness. As you practice further, you can extend this period of stillness for as long as you like. If you hear any external distractions or have any other thoughts that run through your mind, simply use the technique mentioned earlier for handling distractions, and return your attention to the stillness.

When doing this meditation, you should keep a neutral perspective—that is, don't be obsessed with results or "how much energy you generated" or other types of measurements of "success." Otherwise, you'll actually be meditating on the expectations or the expected results rather than on the point of light, the OM, and the intervals between the OMs.

After about ten minutes of stillness, very gently return to your body and move your hands and feet.

8. **Release excess energy by blessing and by rooting.** After the meditation, again raise your hands with palms outward. Imagine

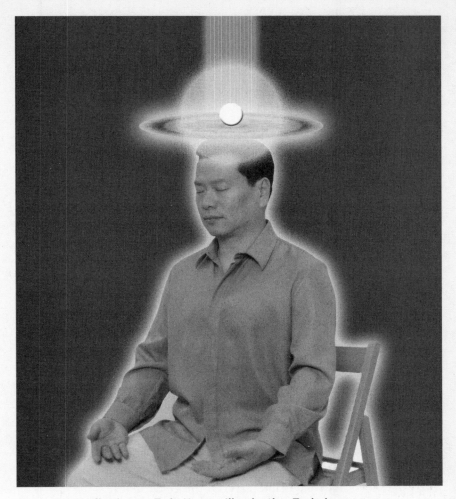

Figure 7.4 **Meditation on Twin Hearts, Illumination Technique**

the earth in front of you again. Release the excess energy by
blessing the earth with light, loving-kindness, peace, and prosperity
for several minutes until you feel your body is normalized. You may
say the following:

> Let the entire earth be blessed with divine light,
> Divine love, and divine power.
> Let the whole earth be blessed with peace, order,
> Spirituality, abundance, and prosperity.
> Let every person, every being, be blessed with happiness,

Good health, spirituality, and abundance.
Blessings be to all.

After releasing the excess energy, you may bless specific persons or your family and friends. Simply visualize them in front of you, and bathe them with the light of the excess energy emanating from your palms.

Next, gently be aware of the base of your spine. Project your consciousness down into the earth, and imagine shafts of white light extending from the sole chakras in your feet and your basic chakra down deep into the earth. Do this for about thirty seconds. Bless the earth by silently saying:

Let Mother Earth be blessed
With divine light, love, and power,
Let Mother Earth be revitalized, healed, and regenerated.
Blessings be to Mother Earth.
I am connected and rooted to Mother Earth.

9. **Give thanks.** After meditation, always give thanks for divine blessings. You may use the following prayer:

To the Supreme God,
We thank you for your divine blessings,
To my spiritual teacher, all the spiritual teachers,
Holy masters, all the saints, holy angels,
Spiritual helpers, and all the Great Ones,
We thank you for all your great, great blessings.
Thank you.

Gently open your eyes with a big, big smile. If you feel some old emotions coming out, that is good. It is part of the cleansing process, so don't try to control or hold it down.

10. **Perform one set of the Nine Energizing Breaths.**

A Few Final Notes on Meditation on Twin Hearts

Here are a few final tips on performing Meditation on Twin Hearts. People may occasionally experience physical shaking or the feeling of strong emotions at various points during meditation. This is typically evidence of energetic blockages being cleared out of the aura as the negative emotions associated with those blockages are being worked through. If this happens to you, or if you encounter any discomfort at all, there are several options. Some people simply continue meditating. Others may stop meditating and perform pranic breathing. Others stop and continue later. Let your personal comfort level dictate your actions.

Coughing during Meditation on Twin Hearts means the solar plexus and heart chakras are being cleansed. Some people may experience what is best described as an "inner explosion of light," particularly during the illumination technique. Although this is quite normal, it can be startling. Again, let your personal comfort level dictate your next steps. You may wish to perform pranic breathing and let the experience proceed. However, if you want to, you can also stop meditating, but definitely root yourself again.

Daily practice yields the best results, but not everyone has the time to practice daily. Try to practice regularly—three to five times a week. If you can meditate at the same time every day, whether in the morning, at lunchtime, or in the evening, you're more likely to produce consistent results. Many people prefer a guided meditation over one that they perform themselves. As noted at the outset of this section, for information on obtaining a Meditation on Twin Hearts CD, see pranichealing.com or yourhandscanhealyou.com.

Prayer of St. Francis of Assisi as "Inner Alchemy"

St. Francis of Assisi is one of the most well-known saints in contemporary religion, and the prayer attributed to him is one of the most widely recited, likely because of the sentiments expressed in the second stanza about empathetic understanding. However, an esoteric reading of the prayer shows that it is also a primer on "inner alchemy," the transmutation of the lower negative emotions, such as anger, fear, jealousy, and hate, into the higher positive emotions, such as loving-kindness for all and compassion for the world—changes that are reflective of an even more fundamental transformation of the energy body. Here is the Prayer of St. Francis of Assisi in its entirety:

> Lord, make me an instrument of your peace.
> Where there is hatred, let me sow love;
> Where there is injury, pardon;
> Where there is doubt, faith;

Where there is despair, hope;
Where there is darkness, light;
Where there is sadness, joy.

O Divine Master, grant that I may not so much seek to be consoled
as to console;
To be understood as to understand;
To be loved as to love.

For it is in giving that we receive;
It is in pardoning that we are pardoned;
And it is in dying that we are born to eternal life.

Alchemy as a physical or chemical practice was the ancient science of changing, or transmuting, base metals—usually lead—into gold. Historical accounts vary as to whether this transmutation was actually achieved, though it was certainly an obsessed-upon topic in every culture throughout the ancient world, and even up until the twentieth century. From European magicians working to create wealth for a king, to Egyptian metallurgists melting down all kinds of materials, to Chinese scholars intent on developing the "golden elixir," mankind has long had a fascination with creating gold from lead.

Throughout the history of esoteric philosophy, however, *alchemy* has referred to a transformation of a different type: the refinement of the energy aura through various purification rituals and meditations. This is a process that seeks, ultimately, to transmute the aura into the "golden energy body," emblematic of exceptionally high spiritual development.

The aura of the average person appears, to clairvoyant observation, as a generally white or bright cloud with a variety of grayish spots in it. These blotches are negative thought forms such as anger, fear, and resentment that we all have to varying degrees. They look like smudges or vortexes in an otherwise shimmering cloud of energy. The more anger, fear, and so on a person holds on to, the more dark spots in his or her aura.

But as a person sets off on a more serious spiritual path, undertaking a life of meditation, prayer, and service to the world, emotional changes begin to take place in the person's personality and energetic changes in the person's aura. Bitterness and resentment give way to mercy and understanding, and the smudges in the aura begin to dissolve. A clairvoyant will see the aura gradually get brighter and then sparkle with gold flecks. The person's spiritual cord—the energetic connection between the Higher Soul, located above the physical body, and the Incarnated Soul, the portion of the Higher Soul residing in the physical body—will become larger and more laced with gold as well. With continued purification, the aura will become even brighter and its gold sheen more dense.

Look at the Prayer of St. Francis of Assisi carefully and see how it talks about replacing "base" emotions and qualities, such as hatred, injury, doubt, despair, darkness, and sadness with "higher" emotions and qualities, such as love, pardon, faith, hope, light, and joy. It's a virtual template for inner transformation and "inner alchemy." Recited as you conduct Meditation on Twin Hearts regularly, the prayer of St. Francis of Assisi is an excellent addition to your daily routine.

DISSOLVING INTO LIGHT MEDITATION

Dissolving into Light Meditation is a powerful exercise that enables you simply and easily to increase your contact with your Higher Soul by helping you "dis-identify" with your physical body. In becoming more aware that we are not all the things we typically think we are—the physical body, the emotions, the thoughts—we come to recognize what we really are: the Soul. In this regard, it is a more basic version of Achieving Oneness with the Higher Soul, an advanced meditation taught in Arhatic Yoga, that, practiced regularly, enhances the connection to the Higher Soul by increasing the diameter of the spiritual cord attaching us to the Higher Soul.

Dissolving into Light Meditation is a multipurpose meditation that works on both the physical and energetic levels, and it works wonderfully with the Nine Energizing Breaths because it generates a lot of high-quality divine spiritual energy that the Nine Energizing Breaths can then infuse into your physical body. It also has a self-healing aspect, as you guide the brilliant energy throughout your entire body, enabling it to cleanse and energize your head, brain, organs, bones, and limbs.

The meditation should take between twenty and thirty minutes, depending on how long you wish to stretch out the final "letting go" sequence—and you can stretch that out for as long as you like.

Dissolving into Light Meditation is suitable for all except women who are pregnant or who think they may be pregnant. As with Meditation on Twin Hearts, the energy may be too strong for an unborn child.

Since there are a lot of detailed steps, you may want to read the meditation all the way through several times to familiarize yourself with it before you practice it. You can also record it and then play it back as a guided meditation.

Exercise 7.2 **Dissolving into Light Meditation**

1. **Cleanse the energy body through physical exercise.** Begin this meditation as you began Meditation on Twin Hearts, with one or two sets of the Cleansing Physical Exercises.

2. **Sit quietly in a chair with your hands in your lap, palms up. Connect your tongue to your palate.**

3. **Invocation for divine blessing.** Meditations always begin with an invocation. You can use the one you learned for Meditation on Twin Hearts, or use the one below. Sit quietly and comfortably with your hands turned upward, resting in your lap, and your eyes closed.

> To the Divine Supreme God,
> To the Divine Father/Divine Mother,
> We humbly invoke your blessings;
> To all the spiritual elders, to the holy masters and saints,
> To all the spiritual teachers and spiritual masters,
> To the holy archangels, holy angels, and spiritual helpers,
> We humbly invoke your divine light, divine love,
> Divine guidance, divine healing energy, and divine protection.
> We thank you. In full faith. So be it.

3. **Inhale and exhale slowly three times.** Don't worry about a special breathing rhythm for this meditation. Just breathe slowly and silently three times, in and out through the nose.

4. **Be aware of your heart, and as you are aware of your heart, imagine someone you love very dearly actually in your heart.** Recall a happy experience you had with that person. Recreate the sights, sounds, and loving feelings of that happy event. Allow your heart to expand with love. Feel your heart center glow and expand as you recreate the loving

experience you had with this person. Feel your heart expand upward . . .
feel the warm feeling moving upward, spreading to the top of your head, to
the crown chakra.

5. **Let the loving energy begin to spread downward through your body.**
    After the loving energy reaches the top of your head, let it begin to spread
    downward from your crown into your brain. Take your time; there is no
    hurry. And from the brain, feel the energy flowing downward . . . spreading
    throughout the face . . . neck . . . chest . . . arms . . . throat . . . heart. Really
    feel the feeling.

    Feel the loving energy continue to spread downward through your torso,
    through the lungs . . . liver . . . spleen . . . stomach . . . intestines . . . kidneys
    . . . bladder . . . gallbladder . . . to all the organs and glands of your torso.

    As the energy filters down, it also relaxes your body . . . every part of
    your body is completely relaxed.

    Feel the loving energy moving down your back and down through your
    spine . . . hips . . . thighs . . . knees . . . feet . . . right down to
    the ground.

6. **Allow the loving energy to continue to flow throughout your entire body.**
    Now move your awareness gently back up to the heart and crown. Be
    aware of your heart and crown simultaneously. Inhale gently and silently.
    Hold it for a second as you become aware of your entire body. Then slowly
    exhale, and as you exhale, be aware of your entire body. Let this exhalation
    carry the loving energy from the heart and crown throughout your entire
    body. Your entire body is getting more and more relaxed as the loving
    feeling spreads through every part of your body.

7. **Allow the loving energy to continue to flow gently into each individual
    part of your body.** Be aware of the entire body. As you inhale slowly,
    assimilate the loving energy into the brain. Hold your breath for a brief
    second; then exhale slowly. Inhale slowly again, and let the loving energy
    spread through the spine. Hold your breath for a brief second; then
    exhale slowly. Inhale slowly once more, and let the loving energy spread
    throughout your throat, chest, internal organs, lungs, stomach, and
    spleen. Hold your breath for a brief second; then exhale slowly. Inhale
    slowly yet again, and let the loving energy spread throughout your
    intestines, bladder, gallbladder, and kidneys. Hold your breath for a brief
    second; then exhale slowly. Inhale slowly, and let the loving energy spread

through your arms. Hold your breath for a brief second; then exhale slowly. Inhale slowly, and let the loving energy spread through your hips, reproductive organs, thighs, knees, ankles, and feet. Hold your breath for a brief second; then exhale slowly. Be still, be aware, as your entire body is filled with loving, peaceful energy.

8. **Begin to allow your body to dissolve gently into the light.** Bring your awareness down to your feet. Imagine your feet dissolving into a brilliant light, a light as bright and white as the tip of a sparkler or sunshine glistening on fresh snow. See the brilliant light move up your legs . . . knees . . . thighs . . . hips. As this brilliant light moves through your body, any kind of physical discomfort or ailment in those areas is also dissolving into the light.

    See the brilliant light move up . . . up . . . up, moving through your midsection. Any kind of illness, discomfort, or ailment in your midsection is dissolving into the light. See the brilliant light move up through the chest. Any kind of illness, discomfort, or ailment in your chest is dissolving into the light. See the brilliant light move up through your arms, your neck, your shoulders, your throat.

    Any kind of illness, discomfort, or ailment in these areas is dissolving into the light. See the brilliant light move up through your face and head. Any kind of illness, discomfort, or ailment in these areas is dissolving into the light. Now, observe your entire body dissolving into beautiful light. As you watch the entire body dissolving, silently say to yourself, "I Am not the body. . . . I exist independently of the physical body. . . . I Am That, That I Am. . . . I Am a being of light." Be still. Be aware. Be aware of the silence and the stillness.

9. **Begin to move your awareness higher and allow your emotions to dissolve slowly but completely into the light.** Move your awareness higher . . . higher . . . above the head and outside the body. Experience and feel a negative emotion you had before: guilt, anger, jealousy, or resentment. Really feel the emotion. Then simply observe the emotion dissolving into the light. The light completely consumes the emotion. As you watch the emotion dissolving, silently say to yourself, "I Am not the emotions. I exist independently of these emotions. I Am a being of pure light and pure consciousness. . . . I Am That, That I Am. . . . I Am a spiritual being." Be still. Be aware. Let go.

10. **Move your awareness even higher and allow your thoughts to dissolve slowly but completely into the light.** Move your awareness even higher . . . far above the head and outside the body. Think of a tangible object: an apple, a car, a house. See it clearly. After you picture it, think of a negative event you had in the past, any negative event. Experience it and see it clearly.

Now, allow both the thought of the tangible object and the thought of the negative event to dissolve into the brilliant light. All your negative thoughts are dissolving into the pure light. Any thought you ever had is now dissolving into the brilliant, pure light. As you watch your thoughts dissolving, silently say to yourself, "I Am not any of my thoughts. I Am observing my thoughts. Therefore, they are not me. I exist independently of my thoughts. I Am That, That I Am." Be still. Be aware. Let go.

11. **Move your awareness even higher and completely dissolve into the light.** Go higher . . . higher. Silently say to yourself, "I Am not the body. I Am not the emotions. I Am not the thoughts." Go higher yet. Silently say to yourself, "I Am the Soul. I Am a spiritual being. I Am That, That I Am." Be still. Be aware. Let go. Meditate on the stillness and silence. Allow yourself to move even higher, to an even more brilliant light far above and outside your body. Silently say to yourself, "I Am one and connected to my higher self, my Higher Soul. I Am That, That I Am."

Allow yourself to move even higher . . . higher. You're dissolving into that more brilliant light. Silently say to yourself, "I Am That, That I Am." Move even higher . . . and as you do, the light gets even brighter. Silently say to yourself, "I Am one with the Divine Spark within me. I Am That, That I Am." As you move even higher, allow yourself to just dissolve into brilliant light. Silently say to yourself, "I Am That, That I Am. . . . I Am a being of pure energy, pure consciousness. . . . I Am one with God. . . . I Am one with all. . . . There is only oneness." You are now observing the observer. . . . Dissolve into the brilliant light and let . . . go . . . NOW. Gently be aware of the stillness, peace, and nothingness. . . . Silently say to yourself, "I Am That, That I Am." You are pure energy with consciousness dissolving into that brilliant light. Let go . . . NOW. . . . You are now dissolving into the infinite ocean of golden light, the infinite ocean of peace and stillness. Just let go . . . NOW.

(This is the final "letting go" sequence, and you can stretch it out and "stay above and outside" your body for as long as you like, or for as long as you feel comfortable. When you are ready to return, continue with the sequence.)

12. **Return to your body; perform blessing, grounding/rooting.**

Gently, slowly, come back to your body, to your normal waking consciousness. Move your fingers and toes slowly. Raise your hands from your lap with your palms facing outward. You will release the excess energy by blessing your loved ones, your circumstances, and the earth. Visualize your loved ones in front of you. Shower them with golden light from your palms. Bless them with good health, happiness, prosperity, abundance, and spirituality. Visualize the people you work with, your job and career with success, advancement, prosperity, and progress. Shower them with golden light.

Next, bless your home, your city, state, and country, showering them with golden light. Then, be aware of your feet and the base of your spine. Let golden energy flow downward from the soles of your feet and the base of your spine into the earth.

As you do this, silently say the following:

Let beloved Mother Earth be blessed
With divine light, divine love, divine power.
Let beloved Mother Earth be blessed, healed, regenerated, and revitalized.
Blessings to our beloved Mother Earth.
So be it.

13. **Give thanks.**

To the Supreme God, the Divine Father/Divine Mother, thank you.
To all the higher beings, thank you
For the blessings of love, healing, guidance, help, and protection.
In full faith, thank you. So be it.

Open your eyes with a big smile.

14. **Perform one set of the Nine Energizing Breaths.**

A Few Final Notes on Dissolving into Light Meditation

Here are a few final tips on performing the Dissolving into Light Meditation. This meditation typically does not cause energetic congestion around the chest or in the heart area in sensitive individuals the way Meditation on Twin Hearts can. But in rare instances, it may. So if you feel congested, simply follow the same instructions offered following Meditation on Twin Hearts.

Because there is a focus on getting "out of the body" with Dissolving into Light Meditation, practitioners can feel a little bit spacey or light-headed afterward if they don't do sufficient rooting or grounding and physical exercises. Make sure you root and ground thoroughly. Massaging and rubbing the body, especially the kidneys and liver area, is helpful, too. As with all three of these meditations, you can perform Dissolving into Light regularly—or even daily, if you wish.

REVITALIZING MEDITATION

The Revitalizing Meditation gives you a quick way to clean and energize both your physical and energy body. It uses three steps and three colors of prana to recharge and revitalize you. As you read earlier, each color of prana has certain healing characteristics that make it suitable for either cleansing or energizing—or both.

In the first part of the Revitalizing Meditation, you use green light to clean and relax the physical body. Green prana has a lower, more physical vibration rate and has strong—but gentle—cleansing power, making it ideal for cleaning the body in this basic meditation. In the second part, you use violet light to clean the chakras and meridians. Violet prana has a higher vibration, which makes it a better choice to clean the more refined portions of the energy body. And finally, after the physical and energy bodies are substantially cleaned of negative energy and negative emotions in the first two steps, you use golden light to charge up and revitalize them in the third step. Golden prana has a much higher vibration rate than either green or violet prana, so it is most effective in settings where the body has already been prepared and cleaned by one or several passes with a lower-vibration prana. Golden prana also makes the energy body more conductive, thus making it able to absorb all types of prana more easily.

As with the other two meditations, women who are pregnant or who think they may be pregnant should not practice the Revitalizing Meditation.

Exercise 7.3 **Revitalizing Meditation**

1. **Cleanse the energy body through physical exercise.** Begin this meditation as you began the previous two, with one or two sets of the Cleansing Physical Exercises.

2. **Sit quietly in a chair with your hands in your lap, palms up. Connect your tongue to your palate.**

3. **Invocation for divine blessing.** Sit quietly and comfortably with your hands turned upward, resting in your lap, and your eyes closed.

> To the Divine Supreme God,
> To the Divine Father/Divine Mother,
> We humbly invoke your blessings;
> To all the spiritual elders, to the holy masters and saints,
> To all the spiritual teachers and spiritual masters,
> To the holy archangels, holy angels, and spiritual helpers,
> We humbly invoke your divine light, divine love,
> Divine guidance, divine healing energy, and divine protection.
> We thank you. In full faith. So be it.

4. **Physical relaxation and preliminary cleansing.** Inhale and exhale slowly three times. As you breathe in and out slowly, feel your entire body relax. Relax your entire body. Now be aware of your entire body, and begin a more purposeful inhalation and exhalation. Let your breathing become slower and more rhythmic. As you exhale, see smoke leaving the pores of your body. This smoke is the dirty energy being expelled from your body. As you inhale, see bright light entering the pores of your body. Exhale stress, resentment, and anger from your body. Inhale light, joy, and peace into your body. Continue to breathe in light, joy, and peace, and exhale stress, resentment, and anger from your body. As you do this, feel your body relax further.

5. **Deeper physical relaxation, part by part.** Move your awareness to the top of your head as you continue to breathe slowly. Your entire head is now completely relaxed. . . . Your face is relaxing. . . . Your eyes are relaxing. . . .Your neck and jaw are now completely relaxed. . . .We keep a lot of tension in our jaw and neck, so breathe into your jaw and neck, and let go of all the tension there. Move your awareness to your shoulders and chest, and let any tension located there be released, as you breathe deeply. Your arms are becoming more relaxed . . .your upper arms . . . your forearms . . . your hands are now completely relaxed. All the organs of your torso and all the muscles of your upper body are becoming more and more relaxed.

Move your awareness down your back as you continue to breathe in and out slowly. Your spine and back muscles are now deeply relaxed. Your lower back is becoming more and more relaxed. Move your awareness down to your waist and hips. Breathe deeply, and as you do, your waist and hips become completely relaxed. Move your awareness down into your legs, and allow them to become relaxed . . .your legs are now completely relaxed . . . your thighs . . . your calves . . . your feet are now completely relaxed. Your entire physical body, inside and out, is now completely relaxed.

6. **Cleansing the physical body in a waterfall of pale, liquid, green light.** Now imagine you are standing barefoot in soft grass in a beautiful field. The sun is shining warmly on your body. A few feet away from you is a mountainside. As you look at the mountainside, you see a waterfall cascading down through the rocks. You also notice that the water is actually liquid green light, a very pale-green light. The pale-green light is luminous, even in the daylight. Gently walk toward the waterfall. As you approach it, step under it, and allow the glowing pale green light to pour over your body. It's a wonderful feeling. The pale-green light is pouring over your head . . . cleansing your scalp. The liquid green light flows into your head . . . cleansing your brain . . . your eyes . . . your nose . . . your ears . . . your mouth. The liquid, luminous green light is pouring over and through your head, and as it does so, it gently breaks up and washes away any energetic blockages in your head. The liquid, luminous green light is pouring over and through your head and down into your throat and neck. Your throat and neck are being cleansed thoroughly . . . the thyroid and parathyroid . . . your voice box. The liquid, luminous green light is pouring down into your shoulders, cleansing them thoroughly and gently washing away any energetic blockages. The liquid, luminous green light is moving deep into your chest cavity. It's breaking down any blockages in your heart . . . your lungs . . . your stomach . . . your liver . . . your gallbladder . . . your pancreas . . . your spleen. The liquid, luminous green light is flowing through your intestines and lower abdomen, flushing away any negative energy.

Now, the liquid, luminous green light is flowing down your spine, cleaning away any dirty energy from your spinal column. The liquid, luminous green light is now flowing through your hips . . . purifying your bladder . . . your kidneys. The liquid, luminous green light is flowing down into your legs, cleansing dirty energy away from your thighs . . . your knees . . . your ankles . . . your feet. Down into the earth.

7. **Liquid green light flows through your hollow body.** Be aware of your entire body as it becomes hollow. Your entire body is now hollow, allowing the beautiful liquid green light to flow from the waterfall through your head and down through your entire body: your face . . . your neck . . . down, down, down. . . . See the liquid green light flowing through your chest cavity with all the glands and organs . . . down through your arms . . . your hips . . . your legs. Down, down, down, the liquid green light gently flows through your spine. Any impurities or blockages are being disintegrated and flushed down through your body and out your feet into the ground below you. Be still. Feel more relaxed. All blockages have been disintegrated. Be aware of how much lighter and more comfortable your body feels.

8. **Cleansing the energy body in a liquid violet waterfall.** You look up and become aware that a few feet away from you is a second waterfall. Gently walk toward it. It's actually liquid violet light. Step underneath it and close your eyes. You feel so relaxed and so receptive. The liquid violet light pours down into the top of your head and into your crown chakra. As the liquid violet light pours into your crown chakra, any negative thoughts and any negative energy is being disintegrated and flushed down through your body.

   The liquid violet light pours down into your forehead and your ajna chakras. Any negative thoughts, negative emotions, or negative ideas are being gently disintegrated and expelled by the beautiful liquid violet light. The liquid violet light pours down the back of your head as well—cleansing the back head chakra of any negative thoughts, emotions, and ideas. The liquid violet light is pouring down into your throat and jaw chakras. Your throat and jaw chakras are being cleansed thoroughly by the liquid violet light.

   Any negative thoughts, negative emotions, or negative ideas are being gently disintegrated and expelled by the beautiful liquid violet light.

   The liquid violet light is pouring down your chest into your front and back heart chakras. It is cleansing them of any negative energy or negative emotions. The liquid violet light is pouring down your chest into your front and back solar plexus chakras. The solar plexus chakras are the seat of your emotions, and the liquid violet light is gently cleansing them of any negative energy or negative emotions. Any anger, resentment, or fear in the solar plexus chakras is being broken up and gently dissolved and expelled. The liquid violet light is pouring into your front and back spleen chakra and the liver on the right side. Any negative thoughts, negative emotions, negative ideas in the liver and spleen are being gently disintegrated and expelled by the beautiful liquid violet light. The liquid violet light is pouring down your body into your navel chakra in the front and the meng mein chakra in the back. Any negative thoughts, negative emotions, or negative ideas in the navel and meng mein chakras are being dissolved and gently expelled.

The liquid violet light is pouring down, down, down into your sex chakra and the basic chakra. Any negative thoughts, negative emotions, or negative ideas in the sex chakra and the basic chakra are being dissolved and gently expelled. The liquid violet light is pouring out into your arms and legs, cleansing them gently and completely of any negative energy. Your shoulders . . . upper arms . . . elbows . . . forearms . . . and hands are being completely cleansed. Your thighs . . . knees . . . calves . . . and feet are being completely cleansed. Your chakra system is now being gently and lovingly cleansed and purified.

All the meridians and energy channels of your body are being filled with this liquid violet light. The liquid violet light is dissolving any negative energy and negative thoughts that have been lodged anywhere in your entire energetic anatomy. These negative thoughts and emotions are being flushed down, down, down through the body . . . through the soles of the feet and into the earth. Now just be still; be receptive. The liquid violet light is pouring down, down, down, flooding your entire body, your arms, legs, and torso . . . your meridians and chakras . . . now.

9. **Energizing and revitalizing in the golden pool.** Inhale and exhale slowly three times. A short distance away, you notice a beautiful pool of golden light. You are drawn toward it. You feel a sense of power, love, and energy emanating from the golden pool of light. Gently walk toward it. Now gently walk in, allowing the soothing golden energy to bathe your body as you slowly immerse your entire body: feet . . . legs . . . hips . . . torso . . . arms . . . neck . . . and then your head. You are now completely immersed in the golden pool of energy, and you feel the power of the energy in the pool as you breathe it in. The liquid golden light is now entering and energizing the chakras of your head: your crown . . . your forehead . . . your ajna . . . the back of your head . . . your jaws.

The liquid golden light is flowing into your throat. Every chakra in your head and throat is now cleansed and energized. The liquid golden light is flowing down into your torso and charging up your front and back heart chakras. Your front and back heart chakras are being charged up and energized. The liquid golden light is flowing further down into your torso and charging up your front and back solar plexus chakras. Your front and back solar plexus chakras are being charged up and energized.

The liquid golden light is flowing down further into your torso and charging up your liver and your front and back spleen chakras. Your liver and your front and back spleen chakras are being charged up and energized. The liquid golden light is flowing further down your torso and charging up your navel chakra . . . your sex chakra . . . your meng mein chakra . . . and your basic chakra. All these lower chakras are being charged up and energized.

The liquid golden light is flowing into your arms and legs, charging them up. Your arms and legs are being charged up and energized. As the liquid golden light enters your chakras, it enters into your physical organs as well. The liquid golden light flows down into your crown and into your brain, recharging and energizing your brain. The liquid golden light flows down into your back heart chakra and recharges and energizes your physical heart, thymus gland, and lungs. The liquid golden light flows down into your navel chakra and recharges and energizes your stomach, spleen, intestines, gallbladder, and pancreas with revitalizing golden light. The liquid golden light flows down into your sex chakra and meng mein. The liquid golden light is revitalizing your kidneys, bladder, and reproductive organs. The liquid golden light is entering and revitalizing your arms, elbows, hands . . . even your bone marrow. The liquid golden light is entering and revitalizing your legs down to your ankles and feet . . . into your bone marrow.

10. **Your body is a sponge absorbing all the liquid golden light energy.** Your entire body is like a sponge soaking in the liquid golden light. This liquid golden light is recharging, rejuvenating, and revitalizing every chakra, every organ, every gland, every muscle, bone, tendon, and ligament in your body. It is simultaneously charging up every chakra and your entire energy body. Your energy body is being recharged by the liquid golden light. So be it. Now, just be aware for

a few minutes of your physical body and your energy body absorbing the liquid golden light. You are now being recharged. As you swim around in and enjoy this liquid golden light, every part of your body is absorbing the revitalizing energy from the pool of golden light. Inhale and exhale slowly. Absorb and store the revitalizing energy.

11. **Emerge from the golden pool recharged and revitalized.** Gently come out of the pool of golden light feeling refreshed, revitalized and relaxed . . . every part of your body feels cleansed, recharged, and revitalized. You are filled with inner peace, joy, and happiness. Slowly open your eyes feeling refreshed, relaxed . . . and rejuvenated.

12. **Return to your body; perform blessing, grounding/rooting.** Now come back to your body, to your normal waking consciousness. Move your fingers and toes. Bless the earth as you learned to do in the previous meditations. Raise your hands from your lap with your palms facing outward. Bless your loved ones, your circumstances, and the earth. Shower your loved ones with golden light from your palms. Bless them with good health, happiness, prosperity, abundance, and spirituality. Next, bless your home, your city, state, and country, showering them with golden light. Then, be aware of your feet and the base of your spine. Let golden energy flow downward from the soles of your feet and the base of your spine into the earth. As you do this, silently say the following:

Let beloved Mother Earth be blessed
With divine light, divine love, and divine power.
Let beloved Mother Earth be blessed, healed, regenerated, and revitalized.
Blessings to our beloved Mother Earth.
So be it.

13. **Give thanks.** End with the same blessing you used with the Dissolving into Light Meditation:

To the Supreme God, Divine Father/Divine Mother, thank you.
To all the higher beings, thank you
For the blessings of love, healing, guidance, help, and protection.
In full faith, thank you. So be it.

14. **Perform one set of the Nine Energizing Breaths.**

A Few Final Notes on the Revitalizing Meditation

While Meditation on Twin Hearts is the basic meditational building block of Grandmaster Choa's system, and Dissolving into Light Meditation helps people begin to experience connection with their Higher Soul, the Revitalizing Meditation gives the novice practitioner a chance to experience some of the higher-level characteristics of advanced meditation—but safely. As noted earlier, it's highly advisable to perform advanced meditations only under the direction of a qualified teacher. But the Revitalizing Meditation allows newcomers to get a taste of gently directing different types of prana through the aura and physical body, a step often found in many advanced meditations. Additionally, the meditation will give you some more practice with visualization and familiarity with the healing characteristics of colored pranas.

FINAL NOTES ON ALL MEDITATIONS

As your meditation practice becomes more of a habit, you may find that you become more diligent in your Energetic Hygiene practice. What's happening energetically is that the prana generated by regular meditators becomes progressively more refined, which means that it has a higher vibration rate and requires a more refined "vehicle"—the energetic anatomy—in which it can be stored comfortably. This typically is a gradual process. What may happen is that you simply find yourself, for instance, with less of a taste for red meat, or a desire to take more frequent salt baths. But whether you find yourself practicing Energetic Hygiene more regularly or not, don't worry about it. Either way, it will be a natural evolution, and your body will tell you if and when it's ready to make such a shift.

One other important tip: don't worry if you can't visualize clearly; don't worry about having perfect mental pictures during meditation. It's more important to conjure up the feeling than the visualization. With steady practice, you'll get better at visualization.

Finally, here's a suggested schedule for daily meditation practice. This presumes using only these three meditations. If you currently practice other meditations, you can work these three in as you like, or as you are able:

- Monday—Meditation on Twin Hearts
- Tuesday—Dissolving into Light Meditation

- Wednesday—Revitalizing Meditation
- Thursday—Meditation on Twin Hearts
- Friday—Dissolving into Light Meditation
- Saturday—Revitalizing Meditation
- Sunday—Off

Chapter 8   Supplemental Energy-Development Exercises

"I've noticed a difference in my energy level since starting the Nine Energizing Breaths," says Jen Pezzani of Missouri. She was in the process of moving and also had experienced some medical issues, so Jen had to reduce her regular medications and cut back on caffeine just prior to beginning the Nine Energizing Breaths. But since taking them up, she says, "I haven't felt as sleepy or tired, and I actually feel more awake and alert. You can actually feel the energy moving through your body when done properly."

The Nine Energizing Breaths are a succinct, focused, life-force-enhancement routine. However, some practitioners often like to augment them with other complementary practices that help push the prana further throughout the energy and physical bodies. Thus, we present in this chapter four more simple, effective exercises that give you some additional options and a way to vary your daily energy-generation routine. These four extra exercises can be added to your daily routine in the places suggested (see later in this chapter and chapter 9), or as you are able to perform them. They're just like the rest of the Nine Revitalizing Breaths: very simple to perform, very effective, very powerful. But the emphasis with these supplemental exercises is less on generating additional energy— though they will do that—and more on assuring appropriate balance and assimilation of the energy in your aura. For instance, the Physical Balancing Exercise and Five Points Energy Distribution help to get the prana into all the "nooks and crannies" of your aura. The Tiger Breath cleans out any dirty or congested energy in your head and upper torso.

And the Ritual of Forgiveness gives you a way to release energy that's been trapped by lingering resentments, anger, and other negative emotions.

PHYSICAL BALANCING EXERCISE

The Physical Balancing Exercise is a very quick way to adjust and normalize the flow of energy through your aura. In fact, Grandmaster Choa said that if he was pressed for time and couldn't do a full routine of Cleansing Physical Exercises, Breathing Exercises, meditation, and the Nine Energizing Breaths, he would just do this exercise ten to twelve times. This routine (refer to figure 8.1 for the sequence of movements) can be performed after the Cleansing Physical Exercises or, really, any time you feel out of balance energetically.

Exercise 8.1 **Physical Balancing Exercise**

1. Stand with your feet about two to three feet apart.

2. Inhale and lean backward slightly from the waist while pivoting your head backward. As you do so, lift your arms in front of you until they are comfortably overhead, and keeping your wrists loose, your hands open, and your palms facing away from you, simply rotate your hands around each other three times in a reverse paddling motion, while keeping your head back (see the first position in figure 8.1). This movement will loosen up both your shoulders and your hands. Throughout this movement, keep your arms relaxed and slightly bent at the elbows. Your back is just *slightly* hyperextended backward. This should be an easy, loosening stretch. Don't hold your breath. Exhale and inhale normally throughout.

3. Next, in one smooth, continuous movement, return your torso to an upright position, bring your arms down past the front of your body, and bend forward from the waist until your fingertips touch the ground just about in front of your toes (see the second position in figure 8.1). (Note: If you have back problems or are inflexible, adjust your posture accordingly. For instance, you can bend your knees or spread your legs wider. This exercise should not cause pain or discomfort. If it does, either make postural adjustments or don't perform this exercise.) Touch the ground at that point lightly, bouncing three times.

4. While still keeping your legs spread, raise up slightly from the waist, then reach back a little farther between your legs, stretching for your

heels. Touch the ground near your heels lightly, bouncing three times. After the second series of three touches, stay bent over but return your hands to near your toes.

5. Staying bent over, pivot sideways from the waist to your left while at the same time touching your left toes with your right fingertips. Keep your arms straight. As you make this pivot, turn your head to the left. Then, staying bent over, reverse the motion, and touch your right toes with your left hand, swinging your head to the right. Swing left, then right, left and then right, for a total of three times each way. This swinging, windmilling movement should be made smoothly but not rapidly. Breathe normally throughout the movement, but you will probably find it natural to inhale to the left and exhale to the right, or vice versa. That breathing pattern also helps you time the movement.

6. Return to the bent-over posture, and touch the ground three more times in front of you, as you did in step three.

7. Next, bending from the waist and leading with your fingertips, bring your arms up from between your legs. Inhale as you come up. As you return to an upright posture, pass your arms in front of your body until they are all the way up over your head. In the same slightly bent backward position, repeat the overhead hand rotations that you performed in step 2.

8. Return smoothly to an upright position. Place the back of your left hand at the small of your back, on the meng mein chakra, and bring your right hand over the top of your head as you bend from the waist to your left. The hand passing over

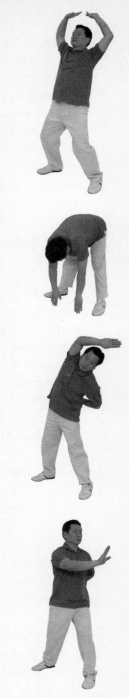

Figure 8.1 **Physical Balancing Exercise**

the top of the head can be either palm up or palm down, though palm up—or away from you—gives you a better stretch. Stretch gently to the left in that posture (see the third position in figure 8.1). Reverse the hand movements, putting the back of your right hand on the meng mein chakra and bringing your left hand over the top of your head as you bend from the waist to your left. Perform this movement two more times in each direction for a total of three times to the left and three to the right. Breathe normally for this movement, but you may find, as you did in step 5, that it lends itself naturally to a rhythm of exhaling in one direction and inhaling in the other direction.

9. Return your torso to the upright position and bring your hands down, but stop in front of your chest. Now twist your torso from the waist to your left, and as you do so, push your right hand as far as you can across your body to your left, palm facing away from you as if you were giving someone a stop sign with your hand (see the fourth position in figure 8.1). Just feel a slight stretch; don't strain. As you stretch your right arm to the left, place your left hand once again on the small of your back, at the meng mein chakra. Now, reverse the motion, twisting your torso to the right and pushing your left hand to the right, while placing your right arm behind your back on the meng mein chakra. Repeat both sides two more times for a total of three times on each side.

10. Perform steps 1 through 9 three to twelve times.

11. Stand up straight and take several pranic breaths.

This exercise should be performed briskly and smoothly. However, as you can see, it has several components, so you may want to practice them separately until you have the individual parts down. Then, you can integrate them all and do the whole exercise in one continuous movement.

TIGER BREATH

The Tiger Breath takes very little time to learn and perform, but it is remarkably effective at expelling dirty energy from the aura, especially the jaw, the brain, and the front and back solar plexus chakras. And because you are expelling a lot of dirty energy, you should perform this exercise either outside or in front of an open window. You can perform the Tiger

Breath after the Physical Balancing Exercise at the end of the Cleansing Physical Exercises. (See figure 8.2 for the sequence of movements for the Tiger Breath.)

Exercise 8.2 **Tiger Breath**

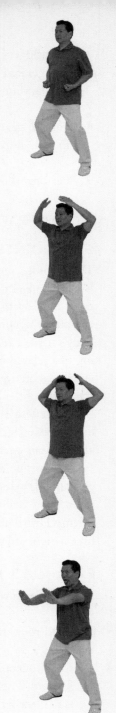

1. If you are familiar with traditional martial arts, this exercise begins in what is called the "high horse stance." This means your feet are a little more than shoulder-width apart and flat on the floor, knees slightly bent. Extend your arms out in front of you, palms up and facing outward. From this stance, take a deep abdominal breath, and pull your hands back toward your body. As you pull your arms in, begin rotating your hands outward and balling your hands into a fist. As you reach the end of your inhale, your fists should be tucked into your sides, just below your ribs, with your fingers and thumbs facing up and the back of your hand toward the ground (see the first position in figure 8.2). Your body should be slightly tense but not rigid.

2. From this position, open your hands and move your arms up and slightly behind your head, almost as if you were cupping them behind the ears to hear better (see the second and third positions in figure 8.2).

3. Now begin to bring your arms smoothly forward from behind your head and past your ears and jawline. As you make this forward pushing movement, begin a slow, controlled—but forceful—exhale, while at the same time rolling your eyes slightly upward, and opening your hands. Exhale with your mouth wide open, your eyes wide open (looking slightly upward), and your tongue fully extended. Exhale your breath with an audible "HAAAA" sound (see the fourth position in figure 8.2). When your arms are fully extended,

Figure 8.2 **Tiger Breath**

your fingers should be stretched wide, as if you are giving someone an exaggerated stop sign. Time your exhale so that, when your lungs are empty, your hands are fully extended.

4. For the next repetition, inhale through your nose, pull your arms back to your sides in fists, and return to the horse stance in step 1.

5. Perform the exercise ten to twelve times.

6. Stand up straight and take several pranic breaths.

FIVE POINTS ENERGY DISTRIBUTION

The vigorous muscle tension and breathing actions of the Nine Energizing Breaths spread the energy throughout the body quite well. If you have a few more minutes in your daily routine, however, you can add another brief exercise after the Nine Energizing Breaths to really drive the prana into all of the body's tissues. It's called Five Points Energy Distribution and involves standing in a relaxed position and performing pranic breathing while keeping your awareness on five key points: the top of the head (crown chakra), the centers of the palms of the hands (palm chakras), and the soles of the feet (sole chakras).

In Chinese Taoist practices, these points are known as the *ba hui*, or "100 lines meeting" (crown chakra), the *lao gong*, or "labor palace" (palm chakras), and the *yong quan*, or "bubbling springs" (sole chakras).

The posture is similar to those used in tai chi chuan or certain styles of chi kung. It's designed to soften and relax the body's musculoskeletal system in order to facilitate the flow of prana or chi. You can perform Five Points Energy Distribution after any other prana-generating exercise, but the ideal time is right after the Nine Energizing Breaths.

Exercise 8.3 **Five Points Energy Distribution**

1. Begin with your feet shoulder-width apart.

2. Bend your knees slightly, no more than a quarter squat.

3. Keep your spine straight, your head up, and your pelvis rotated slightly forward. The best and easiest way to get an idea of what this feels like is to place your back against a wall with your knees slightly bent; then attempt to gently flatten your neck and lower back against the wall. This will lower your chin and raise your head and rotate your pelvis slightly

forward. Don't scrunch your chin down or mash your back against the wall. You don't want to strain. (In fact, your neck and lower back are naturally curved so that it will be difficult to actually place them flush against the wall.) You simply want to stretch out or elongate the spine to enable the prana to flow smoothly up and down your back. A metaphor sometimes used in tai chi chuan practice is to imagine all your vertebrae linked together with a string that comes out the top of your head. If you imagine that you are lifting the string gently,

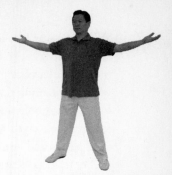

Figure 8.3 **Five Points Energy Distribution**

you can see that you will produce the same effect as standing against a wall: the top of your head raises, your chin drops, and your lower spine slightly flattens out. Try both and see which works better for you.

4. After you establish a relaxed standing position, extend your arms out to your sides, palms up. Keep your entire body relaxed. Your head should be up and your spine straight, but your joints should not be locked, especially your knees and elbows. Your posture should be erect but not tense (see figure 8.3).

5. Place your awareness lightly on the five points: the crown, the two palm chakras, and the two sole chakras. Remember that awareness isn't focused concentration. In fact, it's not a visual sense. It's more that you're simply lightly "feeling" these points.

6. Now perform three to ten cycles of pranic breathing in a 6-3-6-3 pattern of rhythm and retention while keeping your awareness on these points.

As noted throughout this book, the chi follows the yi. When you place your awareness, or intention, on those five points, the energy will be led to them. And since those five points roughly form an outer perimeter of your body, the prana you accumulate during the Nine Revitalizing Breaths will flood your body and your aura.

RITUAL OF FORGIVENESS

It may seem odd to include a forgiveness ritual as part of an energy-development program, but the truth is a tremendous amount of our personal energy supply is tied up in negative emotions such as anger, resentment, and hate.

Why? Because it takes a lot of work, attention—and energy—to hold a grudge and stay angry. The chi follows the yi. And if your yi, your attention, is concentrating on harboring old resentments, a good supply of your energy is tied up with maintaining those resentments, too. Some people have been angry for so long and so automatically, they don't even realize it. But it's easy to tell when you scan their aura: you feel heavy congestion and/or depletion of the front and back solar plexus and heart chakras.

So, to help alleviate some of these negative emotions, we frequently do the following exercise, the Ritual of Forgiveness, prior to meditation. And we do it regularly as well because we're all imperfect, and it's tough to go through life without getting mad at someone or feeling slighted or resentful. It's just one more tool to help you keep your energy supply clean and plentiful.

Exercise 8.4 Ritual of Forgiveness

1. Sit quietly with your eyes closed and your hands folded in your lap.

2. Visualize a person who has hurt you or wronged you in some way. As you see the person, really conjure up the feeling of hurt as you recount what he or she did to you.

3. Now, fold your hands in front of you with your thumbs touching your heart chakra at the center of your chest.

4. With your eyes closed, imagine looking the person in the eyes while silently saying: "The divinity in me salutes the divinity within you." This establishes mutual respect for the spiritual nature in all of us. Then continue: "We are all human. We are all evolving. Evolution means we sometimes make mistakes. Some of these mistakes hurt other people, even if we didn't intend for them to be hurt. I send to you my forgiveness." Pause for a moment, then continue: "God's peace be with you. You are forgiven."

5. Then pause and reflect on forgiveness. Really feel yourself letting go of the anger, resentment, or hurt you were feeling. Smile inwardly at the person.

Repeat three to seven times or until you feel the negative emotion lift. One way to tell if you've truly begun to let the negative emotion go is the ability to think about the person or the original episode without feeling angry or hurt. This is a simple exercise, but practiced regularly, it can be powerful in releasing trapped negative emotional energies.

* * *

These four additional practices will round out your "portfolio" of energy exercises and give you some options for varying your routine. The Tiger Breath is primarily a cleansing exercise, helping you to expel dirty energy from your aura. The Ritual of Forgiveness helps free up emotional attention—and energy—that is stuck because of our inability to let go of lingering resentments. (If you practice this regularly, you will be surprised how much energy you'll get back or recover.) The Physical Balancing Exercise helps regulate your aura. Five Points Energy Distribution gives you another method of making sure the clean prana you generate is dispersed thoroughly throughout your aura. Each has a slightly different use and application, and most people like one or two more than the others. Add them as you have time or are able.

Chapter 9   A Daily Routine for the Nine Energizing Breaths

Catalina Chaw of Southern California began performing the Nine Energizing Breaths twice a day, and felt the effects very quickly. "They really helped wake up my body," she says, "especially in the afternoon. After a long morning and lunch, the body tends to feel tired and crave a nap. But after doing this small set of exercises, I feel energized and ready to go on with my routine. Thanks so much for sharing with all of us."

In any self-improvement program, the key to success is continued regular practice, and that type of commitment to steady training will certainly help you boost your personal energy. Thus, we present here a simple routine to help you build the Nine Energizing Breaths into your schedule, regardless of how busy you are.

Mornings are the ideal time for performing your energy routine because it gives a nice kick-start to your day. However, if your schedule doesn't permit you to have a morning routine, you may try practicing in the midmorning or before your exercise program or even in the evening (though you have to be careful that you don't do the exercises too late in the evening, as they may keep you awake). If you do them in the morning, you should do them after showering but before eating. As noted earlier, water can wash away prana, while a full stomach pulls the body's attention and energy toward digestion and away from building up extra energy. The following daily routine is recommended:

1. **Cleansing Physical Exercises.** One set of twelve repetitions of each exercise. Add a second set if you have time.

2. **Pranic Breathing.** One to three sets of ten cycles of pranic breathing (whichever rhythm you prefer).

3. **Meditation.** If meditation is part of your daily routine, this would be a good place in which to add it.

4. **Cleansing Physical Exercises.** Perform another set to help avoid energetic congestion after meditation.

5. **The Nine Revitalizing Breaths.** Perform one set. You may work up to three sets, as time and your ability to acclimate to the energy permits.

6. **Energetic Hygiene.**
   • Salt baths. Two to three times a week (more if you're stressed out, feeling energetically dirty, or work in a dirty environment).
   • Cord cutting. Cut cords daily, morning and evening. Cut them also as needed to eliminate energetic connection to toxic people or stressful situations in your life.
   • Dietary modifications. Cleaner diet to the extent that you are interested and able.

7. **Midday Pick-Me-Up.** One set of ten cycles of pranic breathing, followed by the first two of the Nine Energizing Breaths.

8. **Adding the Advanced Practices.**
   • Physical Balancing Exercise. Perform three to twelve of these at the end of the Cleansing Physical Exercises or any time you need to get your overall energy aura normalized.
   • Tiger Breath. Perform three to twelve of these after Physical Balancing Exercise at the end of Cleansing Physical Exercises.
   • Five Points Energy Distribution. Perform just after the Nine Energizing Breaths to more fully instill the energy into your aura and physical body.

Consider the above to be an ideal daily routine. You can certainly break it up and perform the elements separately if you're not able to devote the time to all these exercises at once. You can still get great benefit from them individually. After all, it's better to practice them when you can rather than not perform them at all.

Now that you've learned this powerful routine for enhancing your life force, it's up to you to implement it in your daily life. Based on ancient wisdom, but modified and updated specifically for the busy, pressed-for-time modern practitioner, the Nine Energizing Breaths provide a simple, easy way for you to boost your energy and revitalize your body. And when combined with the supplemental practices and meditation (one of the three included here or one of your own choosing), they form a complete program for physical, emotional, and spiritual rejuvenation.

It's a program that we teach and practice ourselves, and we are truly honored to be able to present it to you. We believe these exercises and routines have the power to transform lives, not only by increasing your personal energy supply and stamina for daily living, but also by providing, to those who are interested in pursuing it, entrée to a world of higher spiritual development.

For as you use the Nine Energizing Breaths to heal and energize your physical body, you inevitably—and ironically—come to understand that "you" are *not* your physical body. "You" are something much greater and more ineffable and yet also far more permanent: the Higher Soul.

You come to realize that we are indeed "spiritual beings having a human experience."

Finally, it seems entirely appropriate to close this book with one of Grandmaster Choa Kok Sui's most important lessons, and it's not one he explained directly, wrote about in a book, or talked about in class, but one we all picked up nonetheless. So many of us came to Pranic Healing and Arhatic Yoga initially to learn techniques to be more powerful. Many of us had studied or continue to study martial arts and loved the power behind the techniques. We learned meditations that forced energy into the chakras and caused our auras to be huge. We practiced energy-development exercises that could have kept us up for days on end if we weren't careful about practicing moderation. And we enjoyed the feeling of being "supercharged." But as we continued and matured in our practice, we found out what all serious students of spiritual and energy work discover: the only reason for having all of this energy is to give it back in the form of service. That was the legacy of Grandmaster Choa Kok Sui, that you have to *do* something with all that energy—whether it's healing the sick, blessing the world during meditation, feeding the hungry, or just being present and attentive to your family and friends. That was his most enduring lesson for us all.

And so, along with these powerful exercises, we pass that lesson along to you as well.

Atma Namaste!

Appendix A The Seven Healing Factors and Their Influence on Energy Development

Pranic Healing is very powerful, even miraculous at times, in its effectiveness to relieve physical and emotional symptoms of illness and bring about health and wellness. However, there are certain aspects that affect the efficacy of any healing, regardless of the system or patient. In Pranic Healing, we call these the Seven Healing Factors,[1] and understanding them will make any healing more successful.

We are including information on the Seven Healing Factors in this book on energy, youthfulness, and longevity because they are also general rules that apply to a person's use of prana in any setting, whether it be for healing another or generating prana for your own health benefit. (And if you think about it, what is increasing your personal supply of energy if not self-healing?) Understanding the Seven Healing Factors can help you optimize your Nine Energizing Breaths practice.

1. **Receptivity.** In healing, receptivity refers to the willingness of the subject to keep a positive or at least neutral frame of mind about the healing treatment. While it's fine to maintain a healthy skepticism about any sort of healing effort—either traditional or alternative— unremitting negative thinking likely will not help you get healthy. If you begin treatment thinking "this will never work," or "I don't believe this guy can wave his hands and heal me," then you'll probably get what you're thinking: it won't work, or at least it won't be as effective or long-lasting as it could be.

   Receptivity applies to the Nine Energizing Breaths in much the same way. We don't ask for, nor do we expect, blind belief in the exercises as they are presented here. As noted earlier, Grandmaster

Choa was a stickler for proof, and he urged students to practice what he called "intelligent evaluation." But you should keep an open mind to the possibility that they could work for you. If you're unable or unwilling to give it an honest try and keep negative thinking and negative emotions at bay, you're unlikely to be as effective as you'd like to be.

2. **Skill of the healer.** Healing is a skill, and as with any skill, the more a healer practices, the better he or she becomes. A more experienced healer will be able to draw in more energy, have greater concentration, be more confident, convey that confidence to his or her subject, and thus, likely be a more effective healer. It works that way with the Nine Energizing Breaths as well. The more they are practiced, the more precise your attention to detail, the better you become at the exercises, and of course, the more energy you will generate. This is part of the "energetic compounding effect" referred to earlier.

3. **Severity of the problem.** In both traditional and alternative medicine, the sooner a health problem is detected and treated, the better chance of getting it resolved quickly and completely. If a problem is allowed to become chronic, it becomes more difficult to return to health. Similarly, if before you begin the Nine Energizing Breaths, you're in exceptionally poor health, maintain an unhealthy diet and/ or have unhealthy habits (such as smoking), it may take you longer to reverse those long-term health problems and feel the positive energy-building effects of the exercises.

4. **Age of subject.** As explained, our age is determined by how vigorously our chakras spin and how clean they are. People who are unaware of how to counter the natural aging process through energy exercises and meditation will find their energy dwindling as they get older and thus, may find it more difficult to bounce back from an ailment or be healed by a healer. With regard to practicing the Nine Energizing Breaths, an older person—as defined by the condition of their chakras—may need to practice a little longer and more diligently than a younger person to get the same benefits.

5. **Environment.** Your immediate environment has a huge effect on your personal supply of energy. If you live in a polluted area, eat

energetically dirty foods, and generally do not take care of yourself, either a pranic healer or a physician may find it difficult to heal you quickly and easily. Likewise with the Nine Energizing Breaths: if you keep your body, aura, and personal environment energetically clean, you're likely to make faster progress.

6. **Emotional factors.** Negative emotions such as anxiety, anger, and fear have a damaging effect on your aura, congesting your chakras and meridians and generally reducing your overall energy level. The emotional factor is also tied in with receptivity: if you constantly monitor your symptoms and wonder if each little ache or pain is evidence of the condition getting worse or the ineffectiveness of the healing, your receptivity—and the effectiveness of the healing—will be diminished. The most important emotional factor, however, might be forgiveness, which is really the ability to let go of anger toward someone who has hurt or harmed us. It might also be the most difficult for many people to implement, but it's still very important to work on it—which is why we include the Ritual of Forgiveness as one of the supplemental energy-development exercises. Practicing the Nine Energizing Breaths will definitely help you cleanse some of these strong negative emotions, such as fear, anger, or anxiety, from your aura, but the more of them you have, the longer it may take you to get fully energized. (In addition to the Ritual of Forgiveness, Meditation on Twin Hearts, and The Nine Revitalizing Breaths, there are other Pranic Healing techniques, such as Pranic Psychotherapy, that provide more focused, direct emotional healing. See appendix C for more information on Pranic Psychotherapy.)

7. **Karma.** When a variety of remedies has been tried to heal someone, and the person still is unable to be healed, karmic factors need to be considered. Karma is the cosmic law of cause and effect. "We reap what we sow," and "What goes around comes around," are popularizations of the law of karma. If you smoke and have a diet heavy in fatty foods and then develop heart disease later in life, it's fairly easy to see the physiological cause-and-effect relationship. And as noted earlier, if you've engaged in unhealthy habits for a while, it may take a little longer for the Nine Energizing Breaths energy boost to kick in for you. It's easy to see this as physiological karma, too.

However, many spiritual and healing traditions believe in a much more expansive law of cause and effect: that *all* our thoughts, words, and deeds come back to us in some form or another—either as good or bad health, prosperity, relationships, and so on. In this context, karma may also have a broader impact on your ability to generate energy. For instance, if you're prone to a quick temper, you'll likely have a lot of unresolved anger (negative emotion) in your aura. Or if you have a habit of being condescending or mean in your relationships, this too will fill your aura with negative emotions. And we've already pointed out that holding on to these negative emotions may well affect your practice of the Nine Energizing Breaths.

There are many other aspects of karma, and it's a topic worthy of a much longer discussion. It's covered in detail in higher-level Pranic Healing and Arhatic Yoga classes.

Appendix B Routines and Practices to Increase Energy

T here are many methods that people use to give themselves an energetic boost. Some, such as regular aerobic exercise, provide a simple mental and physical lift. Others, such as more complicated yoga and chi kung routines, are capable of producing tremendous amounts of energy—even to the point of being dangerous to practice without the direct guidance of a competent instructor. And many people combine one or another technique, from this or that system. In this appendix, we offer a brief examination of three of the most popular or well-known of these routines: yoga, chi kung, and tai chi chuan. (Note: These are practices that you can do for yourself, as opposed to those in which you are a passive recipient of someone else's efforts to send energy to you—for example, Reiki or acupuncture.)

YOGA

The popularity of yoga has exploded in the last several years. The 2008 "Yoga In America" study, commissioned by and published in the magazine *Yoga Journal*, reveals that 6.9 percent of U.S. adults, or 15.8 million people, currently practice yoga. Americans also spend $5.7 billion a year on yoga products and classes.[1] Like breathwork, yoga was also listed among the top ten most commonly used complementary and alternative medicine practices in the United States, according to the previously cited NCCAM study.[2]

Most people are familiar with hatha ("forceful") yoga, with its emphasis on asanas ("stable poses") and pranayama ("breath control"), but there are a variety of other types of yoga. Here is just a partial list of the more popular styles:

- Raja ("royal") yoga, which includes intense meditations
- Tantra ("continuity") yoga, which focuses on development of subtle energy
- Bhakti ("devotion") yoga, in which practitioners surrender themselves to God, often through a guru ("teacher")
- Kundalini ("coiled serpent") yoga, which emphasizes enlightenment through development of the kundalini energy at the base of the spine

Additionally, there are contemporary variants from popular teachers, such as Iyengar yoga, a modification of hatha yoga named after B. K. S. Iyengar; and Bikram yoga, a regimented set of postures developed by Bikram Choudhury that is performed in a very hot room.

Regardless of the style, however, since all yogas stem from the same root teachings, a brief history of the development of yoga will yield some of their commonalities. The word *yoga* is from the Sanskrit word *yuj*, meaning to "bind" or "yoke." Thus, all yoga practices—the physical postures, breathing exercises, meditations, and visualizations, as well as the philosophical and ethical guidelines for behavior and conduct—were designed to liberate the practitioner from worldly desires and to "bind" him or her to God. This desired state of liberation and oneness with God, which aspirants may reach after many years of practice, is called *samadhi*.

While the most readily cited written source for yoga is the Yoga Sutras, written by Patanjali around 200 BC, many yogic teachings—and many of the more esoteric elements of yoga—were typically passed down by word of mouth. They weren't put in writing. This is how different types of yoga developed in different areas over its 5,000-year history. A particular teacher would add a certain technique or meditation to his teachings—or perhaps withhold a practice—and that lineage of yoga would be amended from that point forward. Multiply those changes over centuries, and it's easy to see how different types of yoga developed.

But one concept common to all types of yoga is the importance of a guru, or teacher. At lower levels of instruction in more popularized or less esoteric forms of contemporary yoga—for example, a yoga class at your local gym where the principal benefits are physical, such as flexibility and muscle tone—a teacher in the classical Indian sense is less important. For serious students of yoga, however, who have higher spiritual or energetic aspirations, a guru or teacher is indispensable. (While *guru* is popularly translated as "teacher," its true etymological definition would be "dispeller of darkness." Thus, to a spiritual aspirant, a guru is one who cuts through the darkness of the material world and puts the student on the path to light—and God.) Some of the postures, breathing exercises, and meditations can generate tremendous amounts of prana, and yogic literature throughout history is replete with stories of students who, for instance, activated their kundalini energy without proper guidance and had serious problems, including sleeplessness, emotional swings, uncontrolled sexual drive, and many other undesirable side effects.

The physiological and energetic benefits of yoga include:

- **Flexibility and toning.** At a purely physical level, yogas with asanas tone the musculature and promote flexibility.
- **Chakral cleansing.** Since the asanas do provide a real physical workout—indeed, some postures and routines are quite challenging to your strength, balance, and flexibility—they offer the same energetic benefit that all physical exercise does. This means they systematically open and close the chakras, pumping out dirty prana and pulling in fresh prana.
- **"Glandular workout."** Many asanas are designed specifically to massage the lymph system, and to stretch and squeeze the endocrine glands. Improved lymph circulation helps accelerate the expelling of toxins from the body. In many schools of esoteric thought, the seven endocrine glands correspond to seven of the eleven chakras. Thus, exercising the endocrine system helps regulate its secretions, as well as regulate the chakras to which the endocrine glands relate.
- **Direct pranic absorption.** Yogic breathing exercises, together with breath retention and the use of postures, directly draw in prana in a very efficient way.

In addition to an increase in personal vitality and general well-being, yoga practitioners also routinely report weight loss, controlled blood pressure, improved posture, and a more positive, calm outlook on life as some other benefits.

CHI KUNG

Chi kung (also spelled *qi gong*) is a formal term first coined in the middle twentieth century as a way of describing a variety of widely practiced ancient Chinese exercises that generate, balance, and circulate the chi throughout the body. A chi kung style, or "set," typically includes some combination of deep breathing, movements or muscular tension, and intention—and sometimes visualization and meditation. Chi kung has been such an integral part of the Chinese approach to health and well-being that it is considered one of the cornerstones of traditional Chinese medicine, along with acupuncture, herbs, massage, and nutrition.

As interest in alternative medicine and the relationship between life force and health continues to gain wider acceptance in the Western medical community, chi kung, like yoga, has flourished. Chi kung classes are available in many health clubs and other settings. Chi kung is offered as a therapeutic option to cancer patients by the Stanford Center for Integrative Medicine, New York City's Memorial Sloan-Kettering Cancer Center, and the Dana-Farber Cancer Institute in Boston, and is prescribed to those with heart disease at University Medical Center in Tucson, Arizona. Additionally, the effectiveness of chi kung as a health remedy is being researched in clinical trials by the National Institutes of Health's National Center for Complementary and Alternative Medicine for cardiac disease, Parkinson's disease, Huntington's disease, and obesity.

Some of the more popular styles of chi kung practiced today include:

- Wild goose chi kung, one of the most commonly performed sets, in which the movements and postures mimic the movements of the large water bird
- Eight pieces of brocade, one of the oldest styles, which was created by a Chinese war leader to improve the health of his troops
- Tai chi chuan chi kung, another very popular set, which contains eighteen flowing movements similar to tai chi chuan

There are also more esoteric forms of chi kung, such as "iron shirt" or "golden bell," in which martial artists use internal energy and external pressure, massage, and progressively more forceful strikes to their own bodies to make them impervious to physical attack.

Like yoga, chi kung is an ancient practice with deep cultural roots that has evolved over the centuries due to being passed down largely through word of mouth. There are references to chi kung practice in Chinese literature that date back to at least 1000 BC, and there is evidence that breathing modification training took place for hundreds of years after that among scholars and monks. In later centuries, however, many concepts, principally Buddhist, began to trickle over from India, and chi kung began to become more formalized and documented. The Buddhist monk Ta Mo is usually given credit for bringing the physical exercises that were the beginning of chi kung from India to the Shaolin monks in the sixth century. His *Yi Gin Ching* ("muscle development book") has survived to this day.

There were four traditional branches of chi kung: martial arts, in which practitioners built up their energy to make them more powerful fighters (or, as indicated earlier, to make themselves more resistant to an opponent's strikes); health maintenance, exercises to ensure balanced chi flow and well-being; healing, practices to cure health problems; and spirituality, routines to generate chi for enlightenment.

All forms of chi kung, however, share similar characteristics (and these characteristics are similar to yoga, which should not be surprising, given the regular historic migration of thought and philosophy from India to China): modified breathing techniques, various ways of breathing more deeply and holding or directing the breath to certain parts of the body; postures or physical movements, usually smooth, flowing, and graceful (however, some of the fighting forms include swift or dynamic movements); and focused intention, or guiding the chi through the body via the yi, or intent.

The physiological and energetic benefits of chi kung and its methods of producing energy are also similar to yoga:

- **Physical exercise.** Depending on the style, chi kung may or may not provide a significant amount of physical exercise. In some styles, the emphasis is more on breathing, and the movements are minimal or slow and deliberate. Others have more dynamic movements. However, most sets employ some level of muscular tension and relaxation, which the Chinese understood would cause chi and blood to flow into the exercised area. Then, when the muscles are relaxed, the meridians open and allow the chi to flow more smoothly.
- **Opening of the energy channels.** The Chinese speak of meridians and acupuncture points rather than the nadis and chakras of Indian culture, but the correlation between the two systems is evident. Chi kung instructs its practitioners to use perhaps more mental power to move the chi along and balance its flow, but the purpose is the same: to open the energy channels and remove blockages at the key points or chakras.
- **"Internal workout."** Like the asanas, chi kung physical movements exercise areas of the body that are critical to the production of life force but don't get a true "workout" during traditional aerobic exercise or weight training. Some chi kung sets use breathing patterns

that vibrate the organs and glands in rhythm, which exercises and stimulates them.

- **Direct pranic absorption.** Like yoga, chi kung uses abdominal breathing and various breath modifications to increase the efficiency of our ability to draw in energy through the oxygen we take in.

Regular chi kung practitioners cite a list of other health benefits that are quite similar to those reported by yoga adherents: more energy, greater mental clarity and calmness, increased resistance to stress, and greater control over chronic ailments, such as arthritis, high blood pressure, and others.

TAI CHI CHUAN

Tai chi means "grand ultimate," and *chuan* means "fist." Thus, it is a martial art that is the philosophical embodiment of the Taoist conception of the universe, with its dual principles of yin (yielding, soft) and yang (forceful, hard). Together, the yin and yang comprise the "grand ultimate." Like yoga, tai chi has a physical component, and it provides the corporeal body with physical exercise, but its real purpose is to enable the practitioner to transcend the constraints of that body and comprehend the grand ultimate.

Tai chi chuan is an internal martial art, which means that it relies on the development and projection of internal power, chi, which the practitioner converts to *jing*, or "force," to defeat an opponent. This is in contrast to "external" or "hard" martial arts, such as kung fu, which employ muscular strength for fighting. Because it does develop internal power, tai chi chuan is often considered a type of chi kung, as well, and the two are linked together philosophically—and practically. In ancient times the two were frequently taught together, and that is often the case even today.

The story of the origin of tai chi chuan may be apocryphal, but it goes like this: a Taoist monk in the twelfth century, Chan San-Feng, living in a temple near Wu Dan Mountain, developed the physical movements after observing a fight between a snake and a crane. Regardless of whether this or that monk created the movements, tai chi chuan began in the temples and, as with yoga and chi kung, was passed down through the generations largely through word of mouth—either through family clans or in private homes. However, many tai chi chuan historians believe that even within this extremely secretive, closed system of personal instruction, the highest level of practice—which contained many of the true secrets of generating chi, jing, and inner power—was available only in temples.

There were many styles of tai chi chuan, all named after a founder or someone who modified the existing teachings significantly, and most exist in some form today. The original style was *chen*, named after Chen Wang Ting, a general. It is characterized by alternately slow, smooth and fast, explosive movements. It also contains elements of *chin na*, "joint locking." *Yang* style is the most widely practiced today. Its movements are even-paced, slow, sweeping, and flowing. *Wu* style is more compact, with many tight circular movements. *Sun* style is a combination of wu style plus some additional aggressive movements from other fighting styles. These are the basic styles of tai chi chuan, though each may have variations.

Tai chi chuan today may well be the most popular martial art in the world, though most practitioners—at least in this country—seldom think of it as a form of self-defense. Rather, they are attracted to it for the health benefits that many derive from it: improved flexibility, coordination, and relaxation, among others. And it is tai chi chuan's ability to help people reduce stress that has caught the attention of Western medical researchers. Tai chi chuan has been the subject of dozens of clinical studies to test its effectiveness in helping to treat such ailments as high blood pressure, heart disease, multiple sclerosis, arthritis, Parkinson's disease, Alzheimer's disease, anxiety, and depression.

The physiological and energetic benefits of tai chi chuan include:

- **A variety of physical improvements.** Regardless of the style, all forms of tai chi chuan emphasize proper posture and moving the entire body as one unit. The feet are always on the ground, the joints are flexed, and the spine and head are straight but not tense. This usually results in an enhanced sense of balance and integration of mind with body.
- **Calm mind.** The concept of *shoong*, or complete mental and physical relaxation, is essential to proper tai chi chuan practice. Shoong doesn't translate perfectly into English, but it is a very yin idea—that is, the body must yield, or give up. And as the mind relaxes, it becomes more aware of the chi and the body—and how there is no separation between mind and body.
- **Energy flow.** Even if it is true that the highest inner secrets of temple tai chi chuan have been lost, much of the practice today still focuses on developing and guiding the chi throughout the body—with intent. Depending on the instructor, the style, and the diligence of practice, many people can still develop sufficient energy to the point where they can feel it.

- **Direct pranic absorption.** The breathing in tai chi chuan is usually much softer than some of the breathing techniques used in the other modalities discussed here. Nonetheless, with the focus on drawing the breath smoothly and softly to the tan tien ("field of elixir" or "field of chi"), the storage area located just under the navel chakra, tai chi chuan practitioners still engage in abdominal breathing that is very effective at drawing in energy. Additionally, the navel is one of the body's principal repositories for life force in every esoteric energy system. The Chinese systems, in particular, focus on building up and storing the energy there.

Appendix C   Pranic Healing and Arhatic Yoga Courses

Following is a listing of the Pranic Healing and Arhatic Yoga classes currently being taught around the world. Basic Pranic Healing is the prerequisite for all other classes, and it is offered frequently in many cities. For schedules and locations of all classes, see pranichealing.com, or yourhandscanhealyou.com.

BASIC PRANIC HEALING

In Basic Pranic Healing, students learn the fundamentals of working with the aura, including scanning, or feeling the energy; sweeping, or cleaning away congested energy; and energizing, or supplementing areas in the aura that have a pranic deficiency. Pranic Healing has been taught to doctors, nurses, massage therapists, acupuncturists, chiropractors, shiatsu practitioners, and many others in the healing field. All Pranic Healing courses are experiential, which means that students learn by actually performing the techniques and exercises in class—on themselves and other students. And students receive instruction in step-by-step techniques for ailments related to all the major systems of the body. Basic Pranic Healing is a prerequisite for taking all other Pranic Healing and Arhatic Yoga courses.

ADVANCED PRANIC HEALING

Advanced Pranic Healing is a specialized workshop for those who wish to become more effective healers. In Advanced Pranic Healing, students are taught how to utilize colored prana for quicker, more effective healing results, as colored prana creates a more focused effect on the energy field and the chakras. The class includes such advanced therapeutic techniques as rapid healing of wounds, cellular regeneration, cleansing of the internal organs, cleansing of the blood, and a variety of immune-system-boosting practices. Students also learn to enhance the body's innate healing ability to work on serious ailments such as AIDS, cancer, diabetes, and others.

PRANIC PSYCHOTHERAPY

Pranic Psychotherapy is the application of Pranic Healing techniques to remove negative emotional energies and traumatic experiences from the aura and chakras. Students learn simple remedies for healing tension, irritability, grief, and anxiety, as well as how to purge negative programming, usually acquired during childhood, such as poor self-image and various limiting beliefs. Students are also taught to remove the negative energy patterns responsible for phobias and compulsive behaviors, such as addiction to smoking, alcohol, food, and drugs. One of the most significant features of Pranic Psychotherapy is its ability to produce healing results without the patient having to reveal any potentially embarrassing personal information about their fears, traumas, and so on.

PRANIC CRYSTAL HEALING

Pranic Crystal Healing gives students the ability to harness the power of one of Mother Earth's most powerful and precious gifts—crystals and gemstones—which can be used to enhance healing ability, spirituality, and prosperity. The class includes many simple techniques for using crystals to intensify the healing techniques learned in Basic Pranic Healing, Advanced Pranic Healing, and Pranic Psychotherapy, such as activating and revitalizing the chakras, creating personal shields to prevent contamination by the negative or dirty energy of others around you, and using rings, pendants, and jewelry to attract good health and prosperity.

PRANIC PSYCHIC SELF-DEFENSE

The world around us is swirling with thought forms and emotional energies, some of which can be negative or injurious. If we are not properly protected from these contaminants, the result can be spiritual, mental, emotional, physical, or financial damage. Pranic Psychic Self-Defense teaches students how to utilize pranic energies to properly protect themselves and their belongings, surroundings, and loved ones from psychic attacks, negative intentions, malicious entities, and energetic pollution. Students learn such techniques as closing the aura to prevent the intrusion of negative energy; placing a shield around home, business, and financial assets to maximize prosperity and abundance; using the power of love to defuse an angry psychic assailant; and employing holy objects for protection, empowerment, and good luck.

ACHIEVING ONENESS WITH THE HIGHER SOUL

This course reveals ancient meditations that help accelerate the union of the Incarnated Soul (or lower self) with the Higher Soul (or higher self), which is a seed of God's divinity within everyone. This unification goes by various names in different spiritual traditions, including Soul-Realization, Enlightenment, or Self-Realization. The meditations also enable students to cultivate a sense of peace, calmness, and clarity in the midst of a busy and chaotic work or home environment, as well as to experience what is often referred to as the "inner light." The course includes powerful mantras, or words of power, that intensify the meditation experience, expand the consciousness, and increase the size of the spiritual cord, which is the communication cable between the Higher Soul and the Incarnated Soul.

ARHATIC YOGA

The term "Arhatic" is derived from *arhat*, which describes a highly evolved being. *Yoga* means "yoke" or "union." Thus, this advanced yoga system, given to Grandmaster Choa Kok Sui by his teacher, Mahaguruji Mei Ling, provides a powerful blueprint for spiritual development. With origins in the esoteric spiritual systems of China, India, and Tibet, Arhatic Yoga is a synthesis of advanced techniques practiced by initiates for thousands of years that integrates the essence of seven different yoga systems: raja yoga, karma yoga, laya/kundalini yoga, gnana yoga, bhakti yoga, mantra yoga, and simplified hatha yoga. It begins with the purification of the physical, etheric, astral, and mental bodies, after which the chakras are activated in a logical sequence to enable students to circulate the kundalini energy safely throughout the body. This energy circulation technique is practiced by very advanced and evolved yogis and is the foundation for building the much-coveted Golden Body.

HIGHER CLAIRVOYANCE

Clairvoyance is the ability to see the subtle energy, or prana, of the universe. Everyone has the innate ability to see clairvoyantly; it's simply a latent skill that needs to be cultivated. Higher Clairvoyance is a hands-on workshop that teaches students how to develop that skill, which has also been referred to as Heaven Eyes or Buddha Eyes in Eastern esoteric literature. Students learn to activate these specially sensitive "camera lenses" that will enable them to quickly and safely perceive the aura, chakras, and other subtle energies. Those interested in furthering their Pranic Healing skills will learn to use their clairvoyance to more accurately detect unbalanced chakras and areas of congestion and depletion in the aura.

KRIYASHAKTI

Kriya in Sanskrit means "action," "effort," or "deed," while *shakti* refers to creative energy. Thus, Grandmaster Choa Kok Sui's Kriyashakti class teaches students how to properly harness the power of thoughts and subtle energies to create a life of prosperity and success, both materially and spiritually. The class includes dozens of practical techniques, including prosperity meditations to "prime the pump" for abundance; mudras, or hand positions, to accelerate the materialization of thought forms; and a simple method of activating the prosperity chakra to maintain a balance between spirituality and worldly abundance. One key element in the class is a detailed explanation of the esoteric science behind karma, prosperity, and tithing that teaches students how to create their own good luck.

PRANIC FENG SHUI

Grandmaster Choa enlisted the help of numerous high-level clairvoyants to observe the energies of different directions and formations and how they affect health, wealth, and spirituality. The result is a unique class that contradicts some of the tenets of traditional feng shui but also one that produces tangible results. Students learn how to determine the optimum directions in the home and workplace for health, success, and abundance; how to cultivate "prosperity consciousness" by selecting the right colors, pictures, and ornaments for the walls; and how to use the various types of mirrors to capture positive energy and deflect negative energy. The class also includes instruction on "thought power feng shui," which integrates the mind with the immediate environment to positively affect the way people think and feel.

OM MANI PADME HUM

Om Mani Padme Hum is a powerful mantra that generates tremendous love, mercy, and compassion, and in this class students learn the true esoteric meaning of this well-known meditation phrase. Instruction includes using Om Mani Padme Hum to promote true yoga, or union, with the Higher Soul; strengthening the connection with the Higher Soul; purifying the chakras; invoking the Buddha Quan Yin and other wish-fulfilling properties of the mantra; and employing Om Mani Padme Hum as an instrument to bring about world peace. The class also presents in detail how to use this mantra in conjunction with the very powerful Meditation on the Blue Pearl in the Golden Lotus, a meditation taught over the centuries in many different spiritual traditions.

INNER TEACHINGS OF CHRISTIANITY REVEALED

The Lord Jesus instructed the general public with parables, but he gave to the apostles the inner teachings of the "keys to the kingdom of heaven." In this class on the esoteric truth behind many of the symbols and rituals of Christianity, students gain a deeper and more meaningful appreciation of spirituality in general and of Christianity in particular. The class unlocks the true meaning of such New Testament stories and teachings as baptism by fire, water, air, and the Holy Spirit; the Trinity and the three universal aspects of God; the Lord Jesus's washing of his apostles' feet; the Transfiguration; Pentecostal fire; and many of the stories in the book of Revelations.

INNER TEACHINGS OF BUDDHISM REVEALED

The Four Noble Truths and the Eightfold Path as taught by the Buddha are simplified and clarified in this class on the esoteric or inner teachings of Buddhism. Providing a virtual road map to help students systematically re-orient their spiritual and physical life, the class discusses the various schools of Buddhism, the different levels and facets of truth and reality, and the four major causes of suffering (and the solutions to them). Perhaps most important, the class instructs students on how to cultivate the Buddha Nature within you via the spiritual "I," the Atma, and spiritual detachment.

SPIRITUAL ESSENCE OF MAN

Featuring esoteric knowledge and practices from many Egyptian and Indian mystery schools, Spiritual Essence of Man is a unique and powerful workshop that allows students to experience the divine essence within the chakras and energy body. It covers such topics as Krishna's teachings on the Inverted Tree of Life and the Upanishads' Tree of Eternity; the common points in the teachings of the major spiritual traditions, including Taoism, Christianity, Kabbalah, Sanskrit, the Egyptian mystery schools, and others; and the correlations between the Lord's Prayer in the Christian, Kabbalistic, and Egyptian traditions.

SPIRITUAL BUSINESS MANAGEMENT

This innovative workshop uses the immutable spiritual laws of the universe as a template for contemporary business management. Applicable to entrepreneurs, sole proprietorships, small businesses, and corporations alike, these laws help students create a positive organizational environment, increase worker productivity, enhance labor relations, and improve return on investment. While the curriculum is based on ancient spiritual and esoteric principles, the course itself is very businesslike: concise, practical, and results-oriented. It features focused meditations to develop a sharp business mind; spiritual empowerment for management and employees alike that promotes mutual respect, stronger relationships, greater efficiency, and increased productivity; and personal management using the principles of the Seven Rays (human archetypes and tendencies); among other topics.

ARHATIC SEXUAL ALCHEMY

One of the deepest longings of human beings is the desire for an intimate relationship. Arhatic Sexual Alchemy teaches students how to appreciate sexuality as well as create an "energy partnership" to have a truly intimate, deeply fulfilling, and sacred experience with a partner. The class demystifies traditional Tantric and Taoist sexual yoga techniques and enables people to use them as they were intended, while also teaching safe and proper cultivation of sexual energy. Students also learn how to balance sexual energy between pleasure and spirituality, as well as to use sex energy as "spiritual gasoline" to achieve more creativity and access higher states of consciousness.

INNER TEACHINGS OF HINDUISM REVEALED

The format for this class is similar to the Inner Teachings of Christianity and Buddhism classes in that it cuts through superstitions and outward beliefs to reveal the inner meanings and significance behind different deities, symbols, and rituals. The result is a pragmatic approach to understanding the One Universal Formless God through Hinduism, an 8,000-year-old religion. It's a rich class that blends deep understanding of Hindu deities and how and why they're portrayed as they are (for example, why Ganesh has an elephant head and only a single tusk, why Shiva and Krishna have blue skin, why the "perfect disciple" Hanuman appears with a monkey face, and more), with practical application of Hindu meditation traditions, such as the powerful mantras Om Namah Shivaya (used to unlock the power aspect of the Soul), Gayatri Mantra (used for divine guidance, protection, and to awaken Buddha), and Lakshmi Mantra (used to manifest abundance and prosperity).

Notes

CHAPTER 1

1. Grandmaster Choa Kok Sui, *The Origin of Modern Pranic Healing and Arhatic Yoga* (Makati City, Philippines: Institute for Inner Studies Publishing, 2006), 8.
2. Ibid, 78.

CHAPTER 2

1. Grandmaster Choa Kok Sui, *Basic Pranic Healing Instructors' Manual* (Makati City, Philippines: Institute for Inner Studies Publishing, 2002), 13–14.
2. P. M. Barnes, B. Bloom, R. Nahin, "Complementary and Alternative Medicine Use Among Adults and Children: United States, 2007," CDC National Health Statistics Report #12 (December 2008).
3. Jane Spencer, "The Next Yoga: A Sweat-Free Workout—Giving Up on Perfect Pecs, Boomers Embrace Qigong; Tiger Woods's Secret Weapon?" *Wall Street Journal,* May 13, 2003, Eastern edition, Section D.

CHAPTER 3

1. Julie Deardorff, "As Easy As Breathing?" *Chicago Tribune,* June 19, 2005, http:\\articles.chicagotribune.com/2005-06-19/features/0506190439_1_breathing-dioxide-diaphragmatic.
2. Carol Krucoff, "Stress and the Art of Breathing," *Los Angeles Times,* July 10, 2000, Section A, Home Edition.
3. Ibid.
4. Ibid.
5. Grandmaster Choa Kok Sui, *Basic Pranic Healing Instructors' Manual* (Makati City, Philippines: Institute for Inner Studies Publishing, 2002), 59–60.
6. Ibid, 60.

CHAPTER 4

1. Energetic Hygiene material and techniques are adapted from Grandmaster Choa Kok Sui's *Advanced Pranic Healing* (York Beach, ME: Samuel Weiser, Inc., 1995), 34–43, as well as Grandmaster Choa Kok Sui's *Basic Pranic Healing Instructors' Manual* (Makati City, Philippines: Institute for Inner Studies Publishing, 2002), 18, 105.

CHAPTER 5

1. Duke University study, as cited at http://www.dukenews.duke.edu/2000/09/exercise922.html.
2. Eric B. Larson, et al., "Exercise Is Associated with Reduced Risk for Incident Dementia Among Persons 65 Years of Age or Older," *Annals of Internal Medicine* (January 17, 2006) 73–81.

CHAPTER 6

1. Much of the Padmasambhava material is adapted from Grandmaster Choa, *Om Mani Padme Hum: The Blue Pearl in the Golden Lotus* (Makati City, Philippines: Institute for Inner Studies Publishing Foundation, 2004), 2–5.
2. Ngawang Zanpo, *Guru Rinpoche: His Life and Times* (New York: Snow Lion Publications, 2002), 57.
3. History of Padmasambhava from "Padmasambhava," and related entries, *Encyclopedia Britannica* (2003 Deluxe Edition CD-ROM).
4. Account of Edwin J. Dingle's travels from *My Life in Tibet* (Yucca Valley, CA: Institute of Mentalphysics, 1979), 12–16 and 19–33.
5. Original Mentalphysics exercises and related instruction from Edwin J. Dingle, *Breaths That Renew Your Life* (Yucca Valley, CA: Institute of Mentalphysics, 1979), 11–29.
6. Modifications to the Nine Revitalizing Breaths and their effect on personal energy, rejuvenation, and longevity from private instruction and personal interviews with Grandmaster Choa Kok Sui, San Diego, summer 2005.

CHAPTER 7

1. Grandmaster Choa Kok Sui, *Meditations for Soul Realizations* (Makati City, Philippines: Institute for Inner Studies Publishing, 2000), 47.
2. Meditation on Twin Hearts and related commentary adapted from Grandmaster Choa, *Meditations*, 59–72, as well as Pranic Healing and Arhatic Yoga curriculum.

APPENDIX A

1. Seven Healing Factors taken from Grandmaster Choa Kok Sui, *Basic Pranic Healing Instructors' Manual* (Makati City, Philippines: Institute for Inner Studies Publishing, 2002), 48–49.

APPENDIX B

1. *Yoga Journal*, "Yoga in America" study, released February 26, 2008.
2. P. M. Barnes, B. Bloom, and R. Nahin, "Complementary and Alternative Medicine Use Among Adults and Children: United States, 2007," CDC National Health Statistics Report #12 (December 2008).

Further Reading

Choa Kok Sui, Grandmaster. *Advanced Pranic Healing*. York Beach, ME: Samuel Weiser, Inc., 1995.

_____. *The Ancient Science and Art of Pranic Crystal Healing*. Makati City, Philippines: Institute for Inner Studies Publishing, 1998.

_____. *Arhatic Yoga Preparatory Level Workbook*. Makati City, Philippines: Institute for Inner Studies Publishing, 2006.

_____. *Inner Teachings of Hinduism Revealed*. Makati City, Philippines: Institute for Inner Studies Publishing, 2004.

_____. *Meditations for Soul Realization*. Makati City, Philippines: Institute for Inner Studies Publishing, 2000.

_____. *Om Mani Padme Hum: The Blue Pearl in the Golden Lotus*. Makati City, Philippines: Institute for Inner Studies Publishing, 2004.

_____. *The Origin of Modern Pranic Healing and Arhatic Yoga*. Makati City, Philippines: Institute for Inner Studies Publishing, 2006.

_____. *Practical Psychic Self-Defense for Home and Office*. Makati City, Philippines: Institute for Inner Studies Publishing, 1999.

_____. *Pranic Healing*. York Beach, ME: Samuel Weiser, Inc., 1990.

_____. *Pranic Psychotherapy*. York Beach, ME: Samuel Weiser, Inc., 1993.

_____. *The Spiritual Essence of Man: The Chakras and the Kabbalistic Tree of Life*. Makati City, Philippines: Institute for Inner Studies Publishing, 2003.

Co, Master Stephen, and Eric B. Robins, with John Merryman. *Your Hands Can Heal You*. New York: The Free Press/Simon & Schuster, 2002.

Da Liu. *T'ai Chi Ch'uan and Meditation*. New York: Schocken, 1991.

Dingle, Edwin J. *Borderlands of Eternity*. Yucca Valley, CA: Institute of Mentalphysics, 1939.

_____. *Breaths That Renew Your Life*. Yucca Valley, CA: Institute of Mentalphysics, 1979.

_____. *My Life in Tibet*. Yucca Valley, California: Institute of Mentalphysics, 1979.

Farhi, Donna. *The Breathing Book: Vitality and Good Health Through Essential Breath Work.* New York: Henry Holt, 1996.

Hendricks, Gay, PhD, *Conscious Breathing: Breathwork for Health, Stress Release, and Personal Mastery.* New York: Bantam, 1995.

Hendricks, Gay, PhD, with Kathlyn Hendricks. *At the Speed of Life: A New Approach to Personal Change Through Body-Centered Therapy.* New York: Bantam, 1994.

_____. *Conscious Loving: The Journey to Co-Commitment.* New York: Bantam, 1992.

Iyengar, B. K. S. *Light on Pranayama: The Yogic Art of Breathing.* New York: Crossroad, 1985.

_____. *Light on Yoga.* New York: Schocken, 1995.

Kelder, Peter, and Bernie S. Siegel. *Ancient Secret of the Fountain of Youth.* New York: Doubleday, 1998.

Kilham, Christopher S. *The Five Tibetans.* Rochester, Vermont: Healing Arts Press, 1994.

Lam Kam Chuen, Master. *The Way of Energy: Mastering the Chinese Art of Internal Strength with Chi Kung Exercise.* New York: Simon & Schuster, 1991.

Liao, Waysun. *T'ai Chi Classics.* Boston: Shambhala, 2001.

Payne, Larry, and Richard Usatine. *Yoga RX: A Step-by-Step Program to Promote Health, Wellness, and Healing for Common Ailments.* New York: Broadway, 2002.

Reid, Daniel. *A Complete Guide to Chi-Gung.* Boston: Shambhala, 2000.

_____. *The Tao of Health, Sex, and Longevity : A Modern Practical Guide to the Ancient Way.* New York: Fireside, 1989.

Slater, Wallace. *Raja Yoga.* Wheaton, IL: Theosophical Publishing House, 1985.

Yang and Jwing-Ming. *Chi Kung: Health and Martial Arts.* Jamaica Plain, MA: YMAA Publishing, 1996.

_____. *The Eight Pieces of Brocade: A Wai Dan Chi Kung Exercise Set for Improving and Maintaining Health.* Jamaica Plain, MA: YMAA Publishing, 1988.

_____. *The Root of Chinese Chi Kung: Secrets for Health, Longevity, and Enlightenment.* Jamaica Plain, MA: YMAA Publishing, 1997.

Yogananda, Paramahansa. *Autobiography of a Yogi.* Los Angeles: Self-Realization Fellowship, 1993.

Zi, Nancy. *The Art of Breathing: Six Simple Lessons to Improve Performance, Health, and Well-Being.* Berkeley, CA: Frog, Ltd., 2000.

Contact Information

PRANIC HEALING CLASSES, PRODUCTS, AND INFORMATION

U.S. Pranic Healing Center
The American Institute of Asian Studies, LLC
6251 Schaefer Avenue, Suite C
(888) 470-5656
pranichealing.com and yourhandscanhealyou.com

MENTALPHYSICS CLASSES, PRODUCTS, AND INFORMATION

Institute of Mentalphysics
59700 29 Palms Highway
Joshua Tree, CA 92252
(760) 365-8371
mentalphysics.net

About the Authors

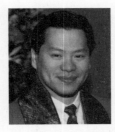

M aster Stephen Co, Eric B. Robins, MD, and John Merryman are the writing team that produced *Your Hands Can Heal You* (Simon & Schuster/The Free Press, 2002).

Master Stephen Co is a personal student of Grandmaster Choa Kok Sui and one of only two Certified Master Pranic Healers in the world. He is a senior instructor at the World Pranic Healing Organization and has taught thousands of people throughout the world including, the United States, Asia, and Europe. He is the author of *The Power of Prana* (Sounds True, 2011) and *Your Hands Can Heal You* (Free Press, 2002).

Eric B. Robins, MD, is a board-certified urologist and surgeon in private practice and affiliated with a major hospital in Los Angeles. He received his MD degree from Baylor College of Medicine in 1989 and his BA in biology from the University of Texas at Austin. Dr. Robins completed his training in surgery and urology at LA County/USC Medical Center. Dr. Robins has received additional training in various alternative healing therapies, including the Emotional Freedom Technique, and newer consciousness technologies, such as Holosync and Matrix Energetics. He is a certified clinical hypnotherapist, a neurolinguistic programming practitioner, and a certified Pranic Healing instructor.

John Merryman is a Los Angeles-based writer specializing in alternative healing, energy medicine, and esoteric and Eastern thought. He has been published in numerous periodicals and newspapers, including *Los Angeles Magazine, California Magazine, LA Reader, Playboy, Cleveland Magazine, Orange Coast Magazine* and the Copley papers, among others.